DIRECT ACCESS TO PHYSICAL THERAPY

THE SECRET REVEALED

How to Relieve Pain & Restore Function WITHOUT Medications, Injections, or Surgery

DR. MICHELLE WOLPOV, PT, DPT, MBA, ATC, CSCS

This edition first published 2017

Direct Access to Physical Therapy © 2017 Michelle Wolpov, Physical Therapy & Fitness By Design, LLC

All rights reserved. No part of the material protected by this copyright may be reproduced or utilized in any form, electronic or mechanical, including photocopying, recording, scanning, or by any information storage and retrieval system, except as permitted under Section 107 or 108 of the 1976 U.S. Copyright Act, without written permission from the copyright owner.

Limit of Liability / Disclaimer of Warranty: While the publisher and author have used their best efforts in preparing this book, they make no representations or warranties with respect to the accuracy or completeness of the contents of the book. It is distributed or sold on the understanding that neither the publisher nor author shall be liable for damages arising herefrom. If professional advice or other expert assistance is required, the services of a competent professional should be sought.

ISBN-13: 978-1975886196 (Paper)
ISBN-10: 1975886194

1. Physical Therapy
2. Direct Access to Physical Therapy
3. Doctor of Physical Therapy

Editing, Layout, and Cover Design: Troy Spinks

For information on quantity discounts or on having the book white labeled for your company, please email the author at: Support@DirectAccessToPhysicalTherapy.com

For Single Orders: https://www.createspace.com/7210327

Printed in the United States of America

"This comprehensive book is packed with useful information that will be valuable, to many audiences, at describing the basis and development of the profession of physical therapy, and the route to accessing physical therapy. Dr. Wolpov has written a detailed resource that explains what a consumer should consider to receive physical therapy, and the benefits of physical therapy to overall healthcare. Given all the recent changes in physical therapy access, and the expected changes to come in healthcare, the timing of this book is perfect. Dr. Wolpov's book supports the vision of the physical therapy profession to transform society."

— **Stephen Lahr, PT, PhD**
Associate Professor and Chair
Department of Physical Therapy, Ithaca College

"All three of my children were patients of Michelle's when they were younger. Not to mention my husband and my father too! And my daughter Lisa, eventually chose physical therapy as her career. Michelle is the kind of person who hopes to make everyone in this world a patient or a Physical Therapist, or BOTH! Physical Therapy has certainly helped my family live more pain free, productive lives!"

— **Sharon Gumnic**
Physical Therapy Advocate

"This book is a breakthrough in consumer/patient education, providing extremely valuable information on the benefits of physical therapy for musculoskeletal injuries and disease. The book is easy to read and understand, and should help answer many previously misunderstood referral requirements for physical therapy."

— **Beth Sarfaty PT, MBA**
Chair NJ State Board of Physical Therapy Examiners
Owner/Instructor Educational Solutions, LLC.

"After going through much suffering and pain from a rotator cuff tear in my shoulder, now I really understand the importance of receiving physical therapy as the first step. Originally, I didn't know about Direct Access to Physical Therapy, so I suffered with pain for 8 weeks while going to my primary physician, then to a specialist, with subsequent delays. Once I arrived in PT, Michelle and her team were excellent at evaluating the cause of my pain, making a clinical diagnosis, and starting treatment the same day. Michelle's book is very informative and a must read for consumers. I wish I read it sooner!"

— **Krishna Ayyala**
Software Engineer IBM

Acknowledgments

A special thanks goes out to the professors and students of Ithaca College, Monmouth University and Evidence in Motion (EIM) for the everlasting knowledge that they bestowed on me. I'm also extremely grateful to my family, friends, and co-workers past and present, for the unwavering support that I received from them over the years. And, to my Mom in heaven, who gave me the wisdom and courage to pursue my dreams.

I also have to give a shout out to David Straight and John Mason from E-Rehab for their awesome websites and social media support; and to Greg Peters of betterPT for his innovative technologies that make finding a qualified Physical Therapist simple and easy. Thank you to Troy Spinks for the editing and layouts of this book. Finally, my appreciation, and a giant hug, goes out to my friend and general manager, Wendy Renzetti, whose hard work and determination allowed me the time to write this book.

#ThinkPTFirst
#DirectAccessToPhysicalTherapy

About the Author:

Dr. Michelle E. Wolpov, PT, DPT, MBA, ATC, CSCS

Dr. Wolpov has practiced in the physical therapy industry for over 30 years. She specializes in the outpatient orthopaedic setting and is a member of the APTA. In May 2002, Dr. Wolpov purchased a local fitness studio, currently known as Game Shape Physical Therapy & Fitness Center in Manalapan, New Jersey. Game Shape is a 5,000-sq. ft., newly renovated state-of-the-art physical therapy facility, which also houses an exclusive one-on-one personal training studio for clients and fitness members. Game Shape is a Rehabilitation Network participating location with the Hospital for Special Surgery (HSS).

In 2005, Dr. Wolpov began consulting as an Expert Witness in the physical therapy and fitness industries. She has handled more than 55 cases for both plaintiff (65%) and defense (35%), writing expert opinions, and testifying at depositions and in court. Her other expert consulting services include: litigation consulting, research and investigation, documentation auditing, independent PT examinations (IMEs), and consulting in standards of care. In 2011, Dr. Wolpov graduated from the EIM – Institute of Health Professions with a Doctorate in Physical Therapy with emphasis in Executive Private Practice Management.

Dr. Wolpov's extensive experience includes providing the most advanced, evidence-based treatment services to patients of all ages, as well as, opening and directing start-up physical therapy facilities throughout New Jersey. Dr. Wolpov has consistently risen through increasing levels of responsibility within the rehabilitation services industry. She possesses almost thirty years of hands-on clinical experience, as well as a wide array of business skills in the areas of: strategic planning, financial management, operations, marketing, quality control, documentation auditing, policies and procedures, human resource management, and business development. She was also recently nominated for the prestigious Athena Award for her commitment to the community and the advancement of women in business. In addition, Dr. Wolpov completed both her MBA and DPT curriculum with a 4.0 GPA and is preparing to sit for the Orthopaedic Board Certification (OCS), through the American Board of Physical Therapy Specialties (ABPTS), in the not too distant future. She has taken over 75 continuing education courses in the areas of orthopaedics and sports medicine.

Table of Contents

Basic Terminology..1
Preface..5
Chapter 1: The History & Definition of Physical Therapy.................9
Chapter 2: Physical Therapy as a Profession.....................................23
Chapter 3: What does "Direct Access Physical Therapy" Truly Mean, and Why Don't YOU Know About It?.......................................31
Chapter 4: Defining the Patient Benefits for Direct Access............43
Chapter 5: The Big-Picture Benefits of Direct Access......................53
Chapter 6: The Military has had Direct Access for Years.................65
Chapter 7: How to Choose the BEST Physical Therapist..................71
Chapter 8: The Case for "Think PT First"..75
Chapter 9: Are PTs Really Qualified to Deliver Services Without a Physician's Referral?..81
Chapter 10: Will There Be an Increase in Healthcare Costs?..........85
Chapter 11: The Argument from Medical Professionals and Chiropractors on Direct Access to Physical Therapy.......................89
Chapter 12: Medicare Beneficiaries - Are You Able to Get Direct Access to Physical Therapy Services?.....................................97
Chapter 13: The Latest Issues That Affect YOUR Rights..................99
Chapter 14: "We The People".... Have Rights!.................................105
Chapter 15: Final Thoughts & How You Can "Pay It Forward".....109
Chapter 16: Your FREE BONUS for Reading This Book...................115
References...117

Basic Terminology

Direct Access to Services: The word "access" in this form means to be able to approach or obtain a service. Direct Access means to be able to obtain a service without having to go through other channels first. In respect to Physical Therapy ("PT") services, it means to be able to see a physical therapist for evaluation and treatment, without first having to see a physician beforehand. It may also be stated as a "Self-Referral for Physical Therapy".

Episode of Care: All services provided to a patient with a neuromuscular or musculoskeletal problem within a span of time across a continuum of care in an integrated healthcare system.

Intervention: An intervention is the purposeful interaction of the physical therapist with the patient/client and, when appropriate, with other individuals involved in patient/client care, using various physical therapy procedures and techniques to produce changes in the condition that are consistent with the diagnosis and prognosis.

DIRECT ACCESS TO PHYSICAL THERAPY

Movement System: The "foundation" and "the core of physical therapy practice, education and research". In a way, it is the "Identity" of the PT profession. The human movement system comprises the anatomical structures and physiologic functions that interact to move the body or its component parts. Human movement is a complex behavior and is comprised of the musculoskeletal, nervous, pulmonary, cardiovascular, endocrine, and integumentary systems.

Physical Therapist (PT): An individual who is highly educated, clinically experienced and licensed to provide physical therapy for the preservation, enhancement or restoration of movement and physical function impaired or threatened by disease, injury or disability, to individuals of all ages. In clinical practice, a physical therapist performs examination, diagnosis, prognosis, and physical interventions through the use of therapeutic exercise, manual therapy techniques, physical modalities (such as heat or cryotherapy, electrotherapy, light therapy and low-level laser therapy), mechanical traction, assistive devices, functional training, and patient education. PTs work in a variety of settings including: outpatient orthopaedic clinics, public schools, colleges/universities, geriatric settings (skilled nursing facilities), rehabilitation centers, hospitals, and medical centers.

Physician: An individual who is educated, clinically experienced, and licensed to practice medicine. This may include, but is not limited to: orthopedists, physiatrists, neurologists, pediatricians, gerontologists, podiatrist, dentists, family practitioners, internists, gynecologists, and oncologists etc.

Profession: A calling or vocation, requiring specialized knowledge after long and intensive academic preparation.

Referral: This word can have several meanings. In this form, it will be used as a noun, i.e. to give a referral. To give a referral would mean that a physician would literally write a prescription for a patient to bring to the physical therapist. Therefore, the words referral and prescription will be used synonymously.

Preface

The purpose of *"Direct Access to Physical Therapy: The Secret Revealed --- How to Relieve Pain & Restore Function WITHOUT Medications, Injections, or Surgery"* is to educate the general public on the benefits of self-referral to physical therapy. It is also to provide valuable information, that until this publication, was primarily shared only among physical therapists.

Physical therapists by nature are caring and nurturing people, who desire to play a role in helping others. Physical therapists sacrifice years to become educated and trained in their profession. Yet, they often lack the skill sets to spread the word, or "promote" what they offer to the public. Academic programs in Physical Therapy typically only offer a few courses in advertising and marketing. Generally speaking, physical therapists aren't looking to become exceptional business people; which is a good thing! I'm sure that you, the reader, only want a physical therapist who is experienced and well-educated in physical therapy, laying hands on you, rather than a professional marketer or businessperson. In my opinion, this is why the information in this book hasn't reached the general public until now.

During the past 25 years, as state-specific direct access laws have emerged, I found myself explaining the rules of engagement, so to speak, of self-referral to physical therapy to each and every person that came into my practice. It was exceptionally rare, that anyone had ever heard of self-referral to physical therapy (i.e. no prescription needed) as an option. Thankfully, I had a gifted way of explaining it to everyone and realized that my practice was becoming more and more "direct access". This meant that the majority of my patients were either coming back on their own when they had another injury or a flair-up of a disease; or they were telling their friends and family about my practice, how they didn't need to see a referring physician first, and those people were coming to see me. People were shocked that they could get right in, that their insurance benefits would cover their physical therapy treatment, and that the entire staff was ready and willing to serve them.

I heard many times over that their experience in my practice, specifically because of direct access, made their lives much easier. Patients didn't need to first wait weeks or even months to see a physician; and they didn't have to spend the extra money on physician office co-pays or co-insurance, and perhaps unnecessary medications, x-rays, or MRIs. Finally, I took the leap of faith to put pen to paper, or should I say fingers to keyboard, so that I could make a difference in the lives of many, rather than limiting myself to only one at a time in my office.

Funny story: I've come across several physical therapists recently who told me that direct access is merely the pathway (the road) to get to physical therapy, and that the general public (consumer) doesn't care how they get there, just as long as their physical therapist successfully reduces their pain and restores their function.

While I highly respect these individuals, I disagree. Here's why: If I'm heading on vacation, I want the path of least resistance. I will inevitably search for the lowest fares, shortest time in the air, with the least amount of stops along the way. I feel that health care is the same way, where consumers will search for the lowest cost, the quickest access, and the least number of stops (number of doctors, pharmacies, labs and imaging centers) to get to where they want (reduced pain and better function).

The inspiration for the book's cover comes from what I refer to as the healthcare "maze". It represents the patient and their families who are getting lost trying to go from one specialist to another, or from MRI to medications to even surgery, without finding the best resolution to their problem. It's my opinion that consumers yearn to find the solution (best option) with the lowest cost and greatest outcome. So, we'll conclude for YOU, the consumer, the road to physical therapy is SUPER important!

DIRECT ACCESS TO PHYSICAL THERAPY

The book is a compilation of articles, research papers, information presented on the APTA website, and other facts and statistics from reliable sources. Of course, my opinions based on 30 years in the industry, 15 of which have been in private practice, all play a role in the book as well.

By reading this book you will learn about the profession of physical therapy, about its long history and the challenges that thousands of therapists have faced to bring about lower health care costs, quicker delivery of care, often with better outcomes to many consumers around the country, by way of "direct access". I'm very proud to be a physical therapist and to have helped so many people in my community. My hope is that you read this book and share it with as many people as you can, so we can spread the word together of what direct access to physical therapy is and the many benefits it will provide for you, your family, co-workers, and friends.

Best in health,

Michelle Wolpov

Dr. Michelle Wolpov, PT, DPT, MBA, ATC, CSCS

Chapter 1

Introduction: The History and Definition of "Physical Therapy"

While admittedly, history is not my favorite subject, I found it essential to write a historical outline of the events that have led us to current day, within the realm of physical therapy. I added some photos, to make this historical rundown more palatable for people like me. For those of you who enjoy history, there are plenty of resources at the back of this book for your reading pleasure.

We could go back in time to 460 BC, when Hippocrates advocated massage and Hector used hydrotherapy (water therapy) for healing purposes and to reduce pain. These were the primitive forms of physical therapy!

In the 1800's, while traveling throughout Europe, Dr. Cameron MacDonald came across archives revealing the origin of the profession of Physical Therapy. Physical Therapy first began in Sweden's Royal Central Institute of Gymnastics (RCIG) and was referred to as "medical gymnastics". Dr. Cameron's research unearthed patient records in which conditions were tracked and manipulative therapy techniques combined with depictive illustrations were documented. Some of these manual techniques, are still being used today (i.e. public symphosis manipulation). Jonas Kellgren, a graduate of the RCIG in 1865, was the grandfather of James Cyriax, MD, who is known as the "grandfather of orthopaedics". Through further research it was found that the Cyriax family continued to promote the growth of physical therapy throughout England in the late 1800's. In 1894, a professional group of nurses in England formed the Chartered Society of Physiotherapy. When traveling outside the U.S., what we know as physical therapy is called "Physiotherapy". If you asked to see a physical therapist, people outside the U.S. may not understand your request, because they are instead referred to as "Physiotherapists" or "Physios"!

The next major countries that began practicing Physical Therapy were New Zealand and the United Sates. New Zealand started a formal training program for physical therapists (Physios) at the School of Physiotherapy at the University of Otago in New Zealand in 1913. Physical Therapy in the United States began in 1914 at the Walter Reed Hospital in Washington, DC. At that time, this hospital was known as the "Flagship" of the U.S. Army, as its leading medical institution. At this prominent medical facility, Walter Reed Hospital graduated the first Physical Therapists, then called "Reconstruction Aides." These were actually nurses with a background in physical education, who were needed to help manage the devastating effects of the First World War (Fig. 1.). The development of the first true hospitals occurred between 1850 and

1900; these institutions were devoted to and organized for only the sick. It was during this time of change that scientific methodology was introduced into the field of medicine. The early 1900's brought formal rehabilitation to the hospital setting.

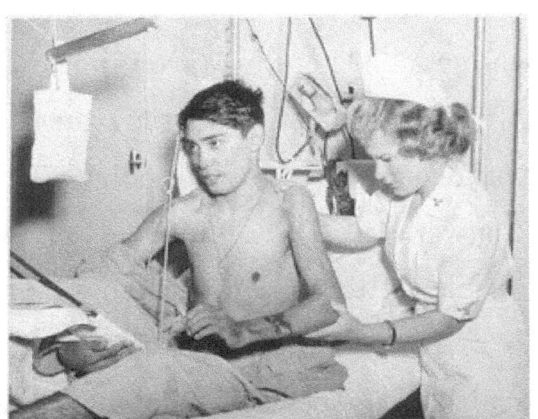
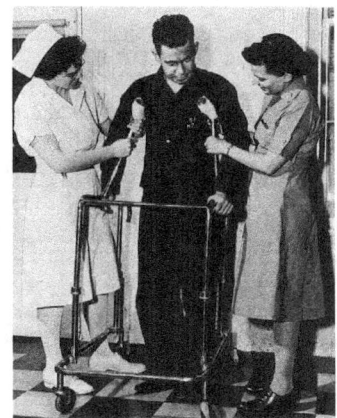

Fig. 1. Early Images of Rehabilitation Aides (Physical Therapists) during the wake of World War I

As with all medical professions, research is a part of the continued development of the field. Research has been a part of the profession since its' early beginnings, noting the first physical therapy research being published in the United States in March 1921, in the first edition of *The PT Review*. During this year, Mary McMillan, PT organized the Physical Therapy Association, which eventually changed its name to the American Physical Therapy Association (APTA). 1921 was a landmark year as educational standards for university professional PT Programs were instituted and programs became accredited by the APTA (Fig. 2.). Scientific research and technology started to shape the profession. In 1924, the Georgia Warm Springs Foundation came into existence with its primary focus on physical therapy for treating the physical deficits of Poliomyelitis ("Polio"), which at the time was a national epidemic. Sister Kenny, PT, who practiced at the Mayo Clinic, was an internationally prominent figure within the physical therapy profession and was well known for her progress with polio. Both polio and physical injuries to war veterans dominated as the primary problems treated with physical therapy for the next 20-30 years. In this pre-World War II era, 80% of physicians were generalists, and only 20% specialized in a specific field of medicine. In the post-World War II era, these figures completely reversed, with specialization dominating most physician's practices.

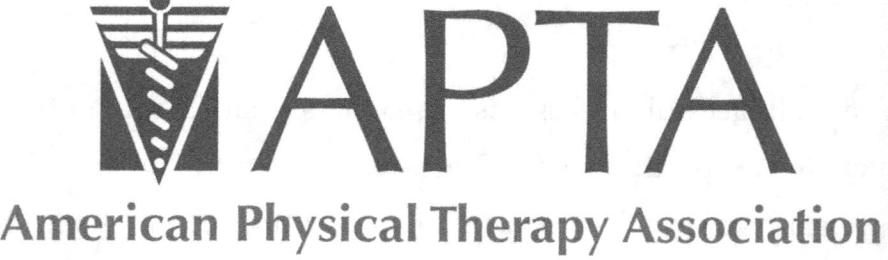

Fig. 2. This is the logo for the American Physical Therapy Association (APTA)

Treatment up through the 1940's primarily consisted of exercise, massage, and traction. Manipulative procedures to the spine and extremity joints started to be practiced, especially in the British

Commonwealth countries, in the early 1950's. During the 1950's, physical therapists began to move beyond hospital-based practice. However, the majority continued to practice in hospitals through the 1960's. Physical Therapists now practice in a wide variety of settings, including: outpatient orthopaedic clinics, public schools, colleges/universities, geriatric settings (skilled nursing facilities), rehabilitation centers, hospitals, and medical centers.

Specialization for Physical Therapy in the United States occurred in 1974, with the Orthopaedic Section of the APTA being formed for those Physical Therapists specializing in Orthopaedics. In the same year, the International Federation of Orthopaedic Manipulative Therapy (IFOMT) was formed, which has heralded change and progress in manual therapy worldwide ever since. During this period of time, the eastern region of the United States was greatly influenced by the training of Norway's Freddy Kaltenborn (Osteopathic Physician, Chiropractor, Physical Therapist, and Athletic Trainer). Mariano Rocabado, PT of Chile, who specialized in treatment of Temporomandibular disorders, also brought much new information and continues to contribute to the profession. Australia's Geoffrey Maitland, PT initially influenced the training of manual therapy on the west coast.

In the 1980's, the explosion of technology and computers led to more technical advances in physical therapy. Some of these advances have continued to grow, with computerized modalities such as ultrasound, electric stimulators, and iontophoresis; and with the latest advances in therapeutic cold laser, which gained FDA approval in the United States in 2002. Other advances, such as electronic resistive exercise known as Isokinetics, have fallen out of popularity for various reasons, despite having a valued place within the profession.

The 1990's brought much attention to manual therapy, with the development of formal residency programs (Fig. 3.). During the summer of 1991, Norwegian manual therapist Freddy Kaltenborne helped create the American Academy of Orthopaedic Manual Physical Therapy (AAOMPT). Dr. Stanley Paris, PT and Ola Grimsby, PT were among the founding members. This organization allowed physical therapists to band together with a common specialization in manual and manipulative therapy. Since this time, formal residency and fellowship training programs have been formed throughout the United States, most of which are recognized by the American Academy of Orthopaedic Manual Therapy (AAOMPT), which is the U.S. national chapter of IFOMT.

In 1992, the University of Southern California initiated the first post-professional "Transitional" Doctor of Physical Therapy (DPT) Program in the U.S. The "transitional" DPT takes into account a physical therapist's current level of knowledge and skill, and offers programs that upgrade clinical skills to meet the needs of the current healthcare environment. Creighton University followed by initiating the first entry-level DPT program in 1993.

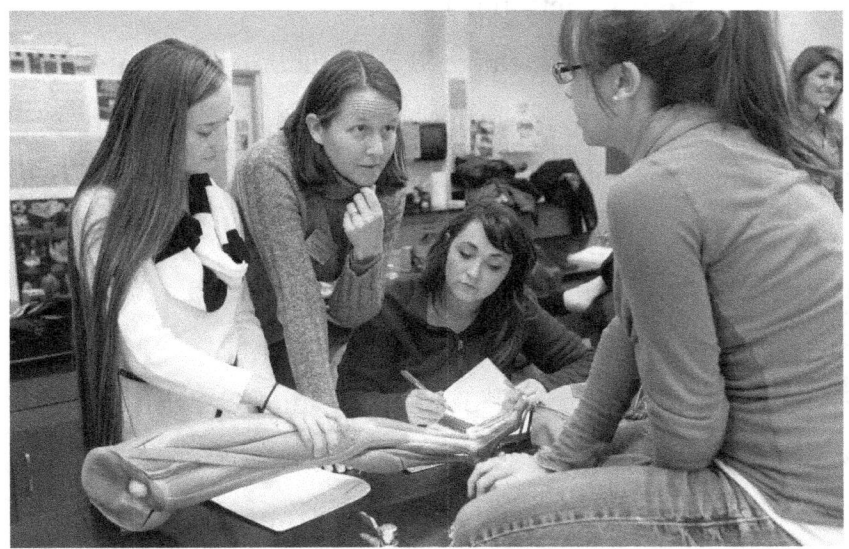

Fig. 3. Residency training programs in the 1990's.

Physical Therapy Interventions

An intervention is at the core of what a physical therapist does. An intervention is defined as: any measure whose purpose is to improve health or alter the course of disease. A more formal definition is, "the purposeful interaction of the physical therapist with the patient/client and, when appropriate, with other individuals involved in patient/client care, using various physical therapy procedures and techniques to produce changes in the condition that are consistent with the diagnosis and prognosis.", as taken from *The Guide to Physical Therapist Practice*.

DIRECT ACCESS TO PHYSICAL THERAPY

Typical Outpatient / Private Practice Interventions:

- Therapeutic Exercises – ROM, Stretching and Strengthening
- Sport Specific & Functional Training
- Neuromuscular Re-education & Stabilization Techniques
- Mechanical Traction & Manual Spinal Traction
- Therapeutic Activities
- Massage and other Soft Tissue Techniques
- Training with Use of Splints or other Orthotics / Prosthetics
- Electrotherapeutic Modalities
- Sports Taping, McConnell Technique and Kinesio-Taping
- Manual Therapy Techniques – i.e. Joint Mobilization, Myofascial Release, Strain / Counterstrain
- Vestibular and Balance Therapy
- Patient Education on Biomechanics, Positioning and Posture
- Low-Intensity Laser
- Instruction in Self-Management to Patient and/or Family Members
- Aquatic Therapy
- Biomechanical and Work-Site Analysis
- EPAT (Shockwave Therapy)
- Activities of Daily Living (ADLs) for Home, Work, or Sport
- Gait Training with Assistive Devices on Level and Uneven Surfaces
- Instruction in a Home Exercise Program

CHAPTER 1

A "Sample" Physical Therapy Treatment Approach:

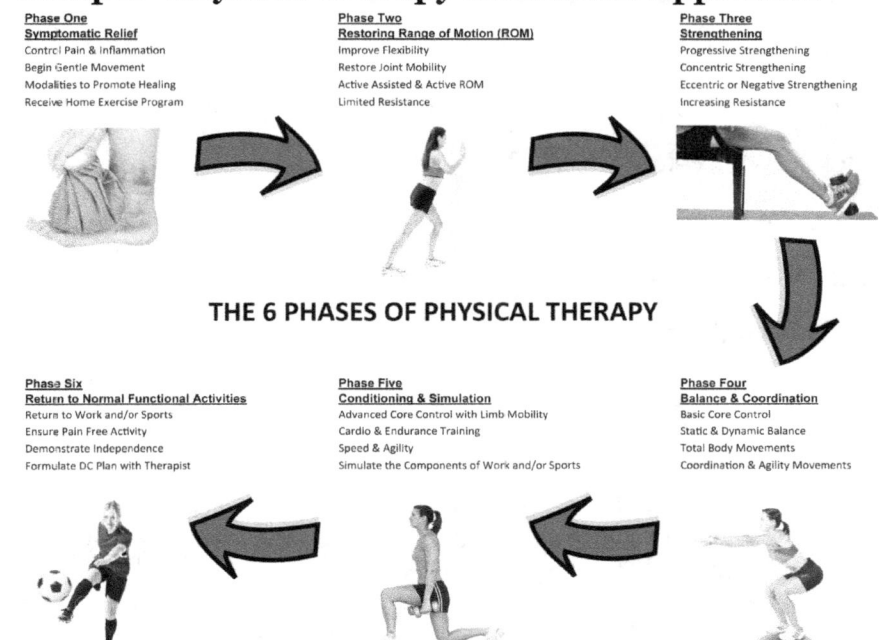

THE 6 PHASES OF PHYSICAL THERAPY

The APTA aspired to what is known as "Vision 2020"

The APTA's Vision 2020 states that, "By 2020, physical therapy will be provided by physical therapists who are doctors of physical therapy, recognized by consumers and other healthcare professionals as the practitioners of choice to whom consumers have direct access for the diagnosis of, intervention for, and prevention of impairments, functional limitations, and disabilities related to movement, function, and health." There are six key elements of Vision 2020, that are elaborated upon in Chapter 2 (Fig. 4.). Despite Vision 2020 being replaced in 2013, this book will cover Vision 2020, as it has made a profound impact on Physical Therapy since the turn of the century.

DIRECT ACCESS TO PHYSICAL THERAPY

The "six key elements" of Vision 2020 are:

1. Autonomous Practice
2. Direct Access
3. Doctor of Physical Therapy
4. Evidence-Based Practice
5. Practitioner of Choice
6. Professionalism

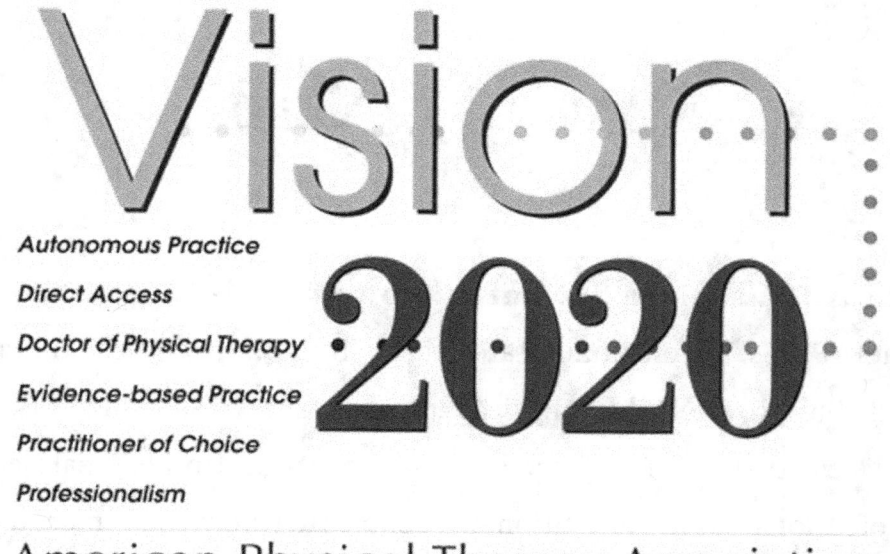

Fig.4. The APTA's Vision 2020 Initiative

The Future of Physical Therapy:

Vision 2020 has served as the vision statement for the physical therapy profession since its adoption in 2000. In 2013, the APTA adopted its newest vision: "Transforming society by optimizing movement to improve the human experience", which is supported by the "Guiding Principles to Achieve the Vision". These guiding principles demonstrate how the profession and the APTA will look when the vision is achieved.

The APTA feels strongly that movement is a key to optimal living and quality of life for all people that extends beyond health to every person's ability to participate in and contribute to society. The physical therapy profession has been called upon to engage with consumers to reduce preventable health care costs and overcome barriers to participation in society to ensure the successful existence of society far into the future.

A Summary of the 8 Guiding Principles are:

- **Identity:** The physical therapy profession will define and promote the movement system as the foundation for optimizing movement to improve the health of society.

- **Quality:** The physical therapy profession will commit to establishing and adopting best practice standards across the domains of practice, education, and research as the individuals in these domains strive to be flexible, prepared, and responsive in a dynamic and ever-changing world.

- **Collaboration:** The physical therapy profession will demonstrate the value of collaboration with other health care providers, consumers, community organizations, and other disciplines to solve the health-related challenges that society faces.

- **Value:** Value has been defined as "the health outcomes achieved per dollar spent." To ensure the best value, services that the physical therapy profession will provide will be safe, effective, patient/client-centered, timely, efficient, and equitable. Outcomes will be both meaningful to patients/clients and cost-effective.

- **Innovation:** The physical therapy profession will offer creative and proactive solutions to enhance health services delivery and to increase the value of physical therapy to society

- **Consumer-Centricity:** Patient/client/consumer values and goals will be central to all efforts in which the physical therapy profession will engage.

- **Access / Equality:** The physical therapy profession will recognize health inequities and disparities and work to ameliorate them through innovative models of service delivery.

- **Advocacy:** The physical therapy profession will advocate for patients/clients/consumers both as individuals and as a population, in practice, education, and research settings to manage and promote change, adopt best practice standards and approaches, and ensure that systems are built to be consumer-centered.

For more information on the APTA's Vision, visit www.APTA.org/Vision/

Chapter 2

Physical Therapy as a Profession

A review of each of the key elements of Vision 2020, is critical to understanding how this development and growth of the physical therapy profession will likely affect consumers (patients) in the U.S. going forward.

Defining the APTA's Vision 2020's six (6) elements:

Autonomous Practice
"Autonomous Practice" essentially means practice without constraints from others. The "others" could be other healthcare practitioners or third-party payors of service. A physical therapist who evaluates a patient without input from any other health care practitioner, designs a treatment plan without any other health care practitioner's input, and re-evaluates the effectiveness of the treatment plan without input from any other healthcare practitioner is surely considered to be practicing autonomously.

Direct Access
Direct Access will be described in much more detail in Chapter 3, but for now, "Direct Access", means that a state's licensure laws would allow the physical therapist to evaluate and treat a patient

without the requirement of a physician's referral (prescription), also known as "physician's orders". There are several different levels of Direct Access throughout the U.S., which limit the physical therapist with certain restrictions.

Doctor of Physical Therapy

There are currently two types of doctoral degrees available in physical therapy. The first is an academic doctoral degree from a university or institution accredited by the Commission on the Accreditation of Physical Therapy Education (CAPTE). The second is a transitional doctoral degree in physical therapy, from a transitional doctor of physical therapy program, that may be CAPTE-accredited. The doctoral programs are referred to as a DPT (Doctor of Physical Therapy) or tDPT (Transitional Doctor of Physical Therapy) program. For the rest of this book, "DPT" will be utilized to infer either type of doctoral program.

Evidence-Based Practice

"Evidence-based practice" means that a patient's treatment plan is based on research that has substantiated a likelihood that the treatment, based on physical therapy evaluation findings, will be the most cost-effective and beneficial treatment. This type of practice means that the physical therapists and physical therapist assistants, must continuously educate themselves and review research for evidence that the treatments being rendered to patients are actually beneficial and effective. In order to facilitate this learning objective, the APTA has an online portal called "Hooked on Evidence" which has evolved into an "Open Door: to Evidence-Based Practice".

Practitioner of Choice

"Practitioner of Choice" essentially means that physical therapists will be the consumer's (or patient's) first choice for treatment of movement dysfunction, dysfunction related to pain, and restoration of function due to diseases and disabilities. There are other professionals who claim to have the ability to also treat many of the same problems physical therapists treat, such as: athletic trainers, massage therapists, exercise physiologists, chiropractors, and personal trainers, to name a few. These other professionals often market their offerings as similar or akin to physical therapy. Thus, being a "practitioner of choice" means the consumer would choose physical therapy services over these other types of service, because of the recognition that doctors of physical therapy are more educated, have greater skills and training, and utilize research to support treatment decisions.

Professionalism

"Professionalism" is defined as professional character, spirit, or methods. The standing practice or methods of a professional, as distinguished from an amateur. The APTA has identified seven "core values" of professionalism in physical therapy as:

DIRECT ACCESS TO PHYSICAL THERAPY

1. Accountability
2. Altruism
3. Compassion / Caring
4. Excellence
5. Integrity
6. Professional Duty
7. Social Responsibility

The APTA has defined each core value and provided sample indicators of the value, which can be found on the Association's website: www.APTA.org/Professionalism/

Since developing a formal Code of Ethics in 2000, physical therapists throughout the country have focused on professionalism, obtaining a higher level of education, providing evidence-based practice and furthering themselves through continuing education. The DPT program has been an integral part of the APTA's continued advocacy for legislation granting consumers (patients) direct access to physical therapists, rather than requiring a physician referral.

More importantly, physical therapists hold a specialized body of knowledge; and as an organized group (i.e. the APTA) the aim is to be self-regulating, free to provide care within the profession's scope of practice, and to ensure that the treatment provided produces an outcome consistent with the best scientific evidence available. With the original goal date of Vision 2020 only a few years away, physical therapists throughout the nation are able to provide some form of direct access to patients and are just now becoming the provider of choice when it comes to treating patients with functional limitations and movement impairments.

The physical therapy profession boasts poised, accomplished, professional practitioners on the cutting edge of healthcare, and it consistently ranks as one of the nation's most desirable careers. In 2017, Physical Therapy as a career is ranked #16, according to U.S. News, and has a projected job increase of 34% by 2024. The increase in job demand is likely due to the growing elderly population, and possibly due to the consumer's ability to get direct access to physical therapy.

To ensure that physical therapy graduates are competent to safely provide evidence-based and effective physical therapy services, the profession has responded to advances in research, technology, science, healthcare, and access to care with changes to the academic and clinical curriculum. Over more than a 100-year period, physical therapy education has evolved from early training programs for reconstruction aides, to its current status, as the doctor of physical therapy (DPT) degree. As of January 1, 2016, the DPT became the required degree for all entry-level

DIRECT ACCESS TO PHYSICAL THERAPY

physical therapist education programs.

According to CAPTE, as of 2017 there are 236 accredited DPT programs with 31,280 students enrolled, and 351 accredited PTA programs with 12,945 students enrolled. Advancement of the profession to the doctoral degree has not been limited solely to the new generation of practitioners. Licensed practitioners with professional baccalaureate, post-baccalaureate certificate, and master's degrees are earning post-professional tDPT degrees. While the tDPT programs will not be around forever, there are nearly 20 programs still in existence. More than 11,000 practitioners have earned a "transitional" DPT degree as of January 2010.

Qualification for licensure includes passing the National Physical Therapy Exam (NPTE) of the Federation of State Boards of Physical Therapy (FSBPT). Another important qualification for licensure is graduation from a CAPTE-accredited physical therapy education program or a program that is in process of being CAPTE-accredited. Physical therapists in the United States are licensed and regulated in all 50 states and the District of Columbia. State licensure is required in each state in which a physical therapist practices and must be renewed on a regular basis, with a majority of states requiring continuing education (CEUs) or other continuing competency requirements for renewal.

CHAPTER 2

As of June 2016, under the American Board of Physical Therapy Specialties (ABPTS), 20,144 physical therapists have been board certified as a clinical specialist in one or more of the following categories: Cardiovascular & Pulmonary, Clinical Electrophysiology, Geriatrics, Neurology, Orthopaedics, Pediatrics, Sports and Women's Health. The majority of Board Certified Specialists remains in Orthopaedics (11,730). In addition, physical therapists have the option to enroll in post-professional residency and fellowship programs, through the American Board of Physical Therapy Residency and Fellowship Education (ABPTRFE) (Fig. 5.).

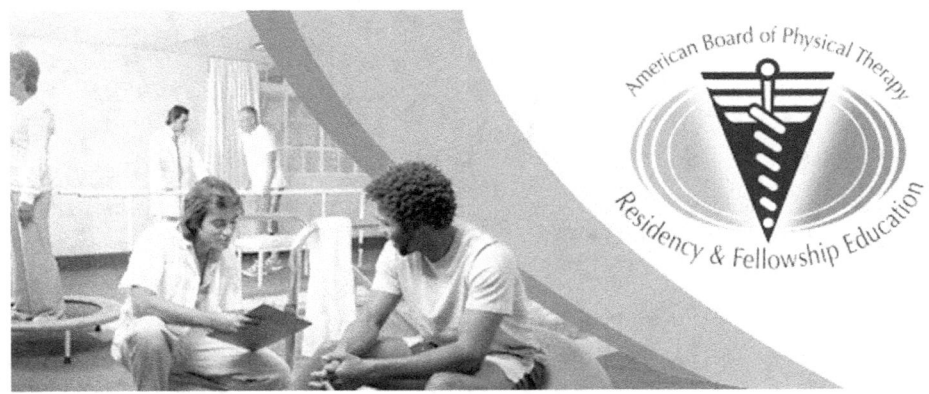

Fig. 5. Fellowship and Residency Programs Emerge

Chapter 3

What does "Direct Access Physical Therapy" Truly Mean, and Why Don't YOU Know About It?

While many Americans are trying to become more conscious of their wellness and physical fitness, there is still a major challenge with the escalating cost of healthcare services. There is growing pressure from the federal government, insurance companies, employers, and the patients themselves for high quality healthcare to be delivered more cost effectively. Since the 1990's, state legislatures have been supporting reforms on the healthcare system. In this regard, focus has been shifted to two key areas: increasing access to healthcare services and containing healthcare costs.

Prior to the 1990's, the practice of physical therapy was stringently regulated in all states. During this period, a patient could only receive physical therapy treatment with a physician's referral (a prescription), which implicitly "cleared" the patient for physical therapy services. In other cases, the physician would have to sign the plan of care written by the physical therapist, in order for the physical therapist to legally deliver the physical therapy treatment. In these situations, the physician was responsible for the overall services delivered to the patient pursuant to the prescription. The physical therapist would simply comply with the specific orders listed on the prescription. If the physical therapist wanted to modify, remove, or add a treatment, they would have to get written approval from the referring physician.

This schematic of liability/responsibility was attractive to physical therapists, as they would essentially have less liability risk, as it would fall primarily on the physician. In fact, there are cases that discuss situations involving a physical therapist or physical therapist assistant, wherein the therapist was not even named as a defendant, meaning the burden fell solely on the referring physician. Early on physical therapists weren't required to carry malpractice (liability) insurance. Even when the physical therapist did carry liability coverage, it was minimal in comparison to the physician. Plaintiff attorneys, also preferred this scenario, because the greater amounts of insurance carried by physicians, meant larger settlements.

During the 1990's, when physical therapists began obtaining Master's Degrees, as opposed to Bachelor's Degrees, it became more common practice for physicians to simply prescribe: "Evaluate and Treat as indicated". Thus, physicians were no longer dictating specifically what the physical therapists should do with a patient, but rather leaving the evaluation and treatment decisions to the knowledge, judgment, and discretion of the physical therapists.

CHAPTER 3

This growth and elevated responsibility of the physical therapist in patient care led the APTA to develop a cohesive direction for the profession, by using the previously covered vision statement known as "Vision 2020". Vision 2020 was the APTA's global goal, ultimately to answer the question: "What will success look like for this organization (profession)?" With the year 2020 rapidly approaching, the APTA has fostered changes to ensure that all physical therapists and physical therapist assistants renew their commitment to the profession, are highly educated at the doctorate level, have a thorough understanding of "direct access" and know how to provide cost-effective, evidence-based treatments.

With the 8 Guiding Principles and the newly adopted Vision, the APTA is now committed to helping physical therapists engage with consumers to reduce preventable healthcare costs, and to overcoming the barriers to physical therapy care that will allow

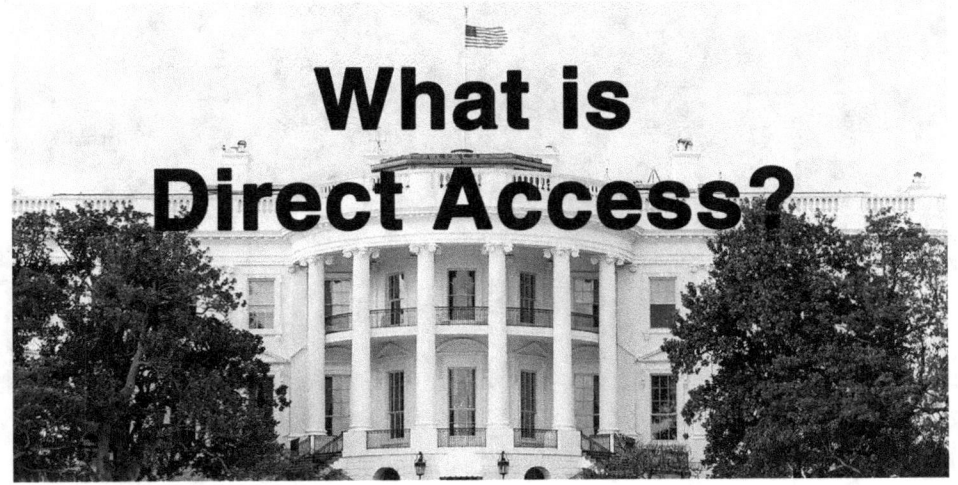

physical therapists to optimize human movement and improve every person's experience in society.

What does "Direct Access to Physical Therapy" really mean? As defined earlier in this book, Direct Access means the removal of the requirement that a physician had to refer (by writing a prescription) a patient to physical therapy, in order for the patient to legally be seen by the physical therapist (Fig. 6.). Direct Access is governed by state laws within the state's "Physical Therapy Practice Act".

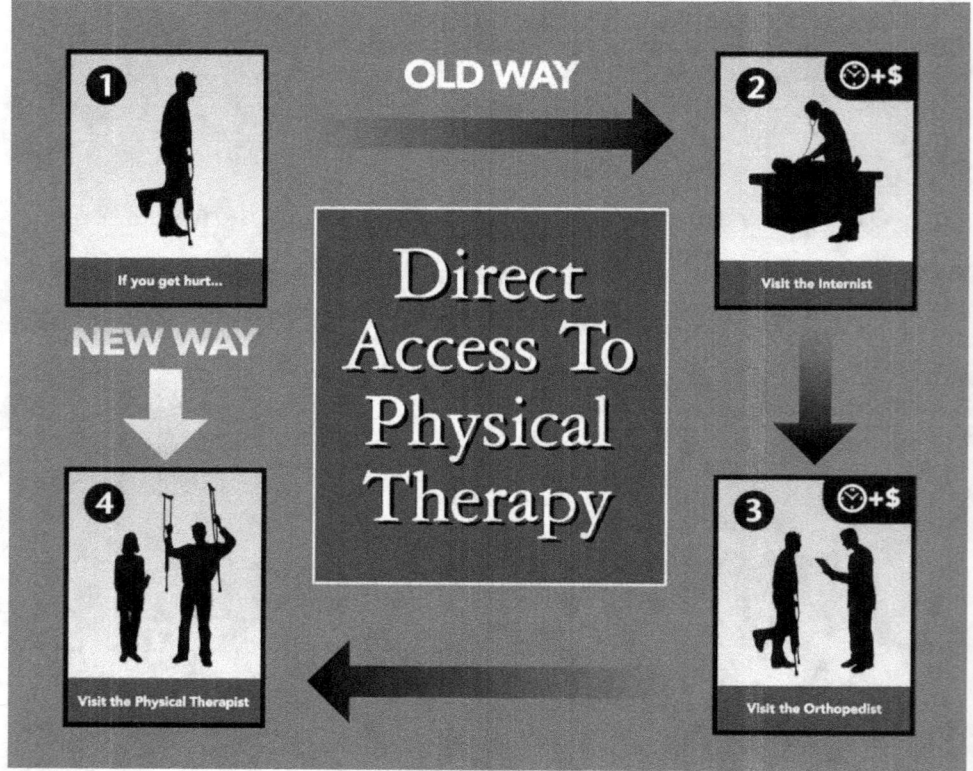

Fig. 6. A Schematic explaining Direct Access to Physical Therapy

CHAPTER 3

Based on data from the APTA, Nebraska was the first state to have some form of direct access, which occurred in 1957. Unfortunately, it has been a multi-decade struggle to achieve direct access in every state. Given fierce opposition from physician groups, chiropractors, and others, APTA leaders at the state level had to fight to alleviate access restrictions. Each small win achieved by the APTA was used as momentum for further policy changes. The first step was to start with small changes in the states' laws. A huge victory was finally achieved in 1991, when Texas physical therapists won the right to evaluate patients without a referral.

The triumphs often fell short of giving consumers "unrestricted" patient access to physical therapy services. It wasn't until the 2000's that several state chapters waged successful fights to further liberate that access. The political process required negotiation, patience and compromise; and this resulted in a patchwork of direct access laws across the country. By the end of 2013, Oklahoma and Michigan became the 49th and 50th states to get on the list of direct access states. This was truly the work of thousands of physical therapists to make direct access a reality on behalf of the patients.

By 2014, every state in the U.S., the District of Columbia and the U.S. Virgin Islands, allowed for the evaluation and some form of treatment without physician referral. As of 2016, there was "unrestricted" patient access in 18 states. That is defined by the

DIRECT ACCESS TO PHYSICAL THERAPY

APTA as "no restrictions or limitations whatsoever for treatment absent a referral". While there is still much work to be done by the physical therapists and physical therapist assistants within the APTA, their achievement in the legal movement for patient's rights to have direct access to physical therapy services has been successful.

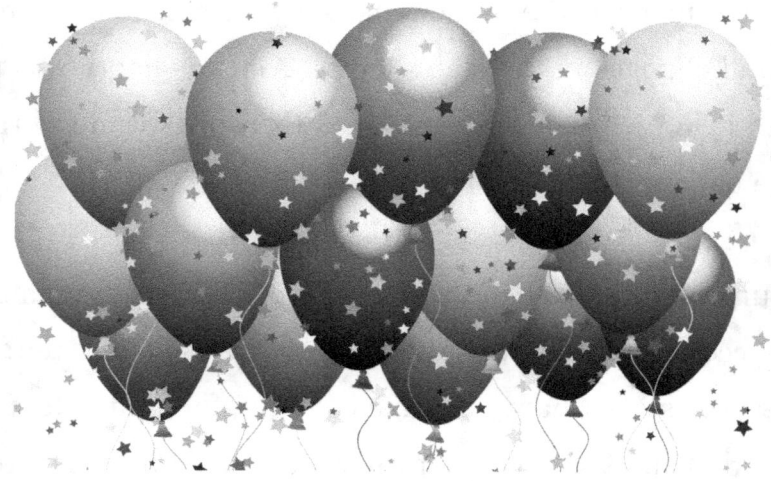

So, congratulations! Finally, everyone in the U.S. is able to receive some form of direct access to physical therapy! While there are still states that impose arbitrary restrictions, which is covered in Chapter 13, for now, it's a celebration and you're invited.

The sad fact is, that the majority of Americans have not received their party invitations and still believe that they must first obtain a referral (prescription), from a physician to see a physical therapist. Even in this day and age, when I visit with medical doctors and surgeons, it is very common that they still believe that

CHAPTER 3

a prescription must come from them, for their own patients to see a physical therapist, as if they are the gatekeepers for physical therapy referrals. Hello! This is simply NOT true anymore!

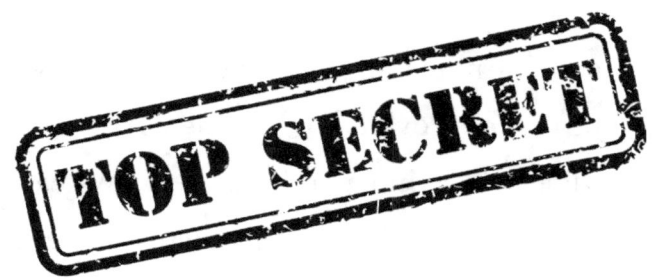

This is the BIGGEST KEPT SECRET to your musculoskeletal health and well-being! Only a fraction of the population realizes that there is a law known as "Direct Access to Physical Therapy" within their state's Physical Therapy Practice Act. Why don't you know about Direct Access to Physical Therapy? Isn't this the age of text messaging and social media? You might ask this very question and the answer is surprising!

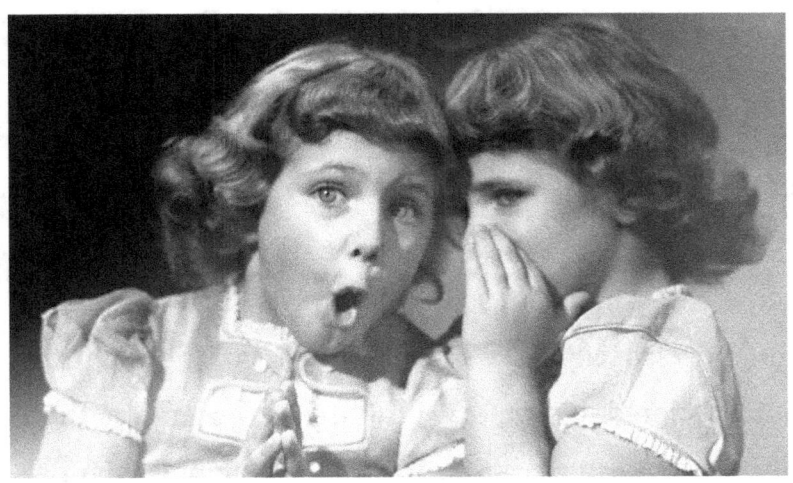

DIRECT ACCESS TO PHYSICAL THERAPY

First, physical therapists realized that with Direct Access, came greater rules and requirements for properly documenting their patient notes. When it came to commercial health insurance, the manner in which PTs were legally allowed to provide direct access service and document notes, unfortunately didn't align with what they were required to provide for payment. Every commercial insurance provider was independent, so physical therapists were forced to check both their state's practice act and with each insurance carrier's billing requirements in order to ensure proper documentation.

Second, physical therapists in many states are unable to order x-rays, MRIs and the like, so they must rely on their clinical evaluation and clinical decision-making skills to identify patients who might not be physical therapy candidates (called "differential diagnosing"), and refer them to the appropriate care providers. Hence, documentation also needed to demonstrate how the physical therapist arrived at their treatment diagnosis and explain how they ruled out other diagnoses. Until the training of differential diagnosing finally caught up with the laws, and non-doctorate physical therapists received the training and developed the competency, many physical therapists in that situation were nervous about the liability risks. Thus, some physical therapists consciously decided not to allow direct access in their clinic and preferred to still get a prescription from a physician.

CHAPTER 3

Third, when direct access first came about, many physical therapists were afraid of telling the general public (consumers) about self-referral to physical therapy, because PTs believed their liability (malpractice) insurance rates would increase if they saw patients through direct access! Physical therapists had typically paid $300 - $500 annually for individual malpractice (liability) coverage, with their physician counterparts paying on average of $18,000 - $20,000 depending on their specialty, and orthopaedic surgeons paying a whopping $25,000/year.

It is still difficult to know the impact of direct access on liability claims, because most states with direct access still to this day have some form of physician control over the services, and not all practicing physical therapists and physical therapist assistants carry malpractice insurance. Hence, if a physical therapist or physical therapist assistant is sued and has no professional liability insurance, the likelihood that the claim would be reported for tracking statistics is slim to none. Yet, the company that the physical therapist is employed by, will most certainly have coverage. The liability aspect is an area that is closely monitored, but to date, insurance rates have not risen significantly as once feared.

However, physical therapists, physical therapist assistants, and students should read any opinions that professional malpractice claims have not risen as a result of direct access to physical therapy with some skepticism. Through Health Providers Service Organization (HPSO), CNA continues to be the nation's largest underwriter of professional liability insurance coverage for physical therapists, with over 79,000 policies in force since 2016. According to the most recent CNA report (2016), in the years spanning from 2000 – 2010, physical therapy liability claims averaged 48 claims/year. However, data taken from 2011 – 2015, showed an increase in annual claims averaging 89 claims/year, which is nearly twice as many. Again, this could be due in part to the increase in the number of insured physical therapists or the number of patients now receiving physical therapy. Consequently, this would explain why physical therapists were initially resistant to direct access.

Fourth, while almost all physical therapists across the nation know about the direct access laws in their state, it is admittedly very difficult to get the word out. Typically, physical therapy companies will have a small section about direct access on their websites and perhaps a blog or two. Spreading the word about direct access to physical therapy is hard work. Most physical therapists are only offered one or two classes in practice management, entrepreneurship or marketing. It takes a lot of creativity and time to reach consumers with any offer of a product or service, even if it is beneficial to majority of people. Most physical therapists find that having direct access leads to greater competition in the industry and they find themselves spending even more time trying to figure ways of differentiating themselves.

Finally, another reason that physical therapists might be leery to hang out a shingle saying "direct access" is they're afraid that referring physicians would stop referring to them. For decades, physicians were the gatekeepers to physical therapy. They were the major source of new patients coming in for physical therapy. In many places, this is still the case. Physical therapists would market to physicians like they were pharmaceutical reps distributing samples of new medications. They relied heavily on these physician referrals. Physical therapists worried that if physicians believed that physical therapists didn't need them anymore, then the physicians would simply stop referring.

In my opinion, physical therapists were unsure of their own ability to market directly to the consumer utilizing direct access and they did not want to sever the lifeblood of their business, the physicians. In addition, marketing to a limited number of physicians is certainly less expensive than marketing to the general public. The APTA has spent a lot of time and money on putting their efforts into educating physical therapists on how to market, or what I call, "spreading valuable information" about Direct Access. Thankfully, physical therapists are learning that they can survive without relying on physician referrals, but it has taken decades.

Chapter 4

Defining the Patient Benefits for Direct Access Physical Therapy

Let's breakdown the benefits of direct access physical therapy into two distinct categories:

Patient-Centric Benefits: Benefits that deal with the individual consumer's choice of convenience and level of control.

Global Benefits: Benefits that help lower costs and improve healthcare at the local, state, and national levels.

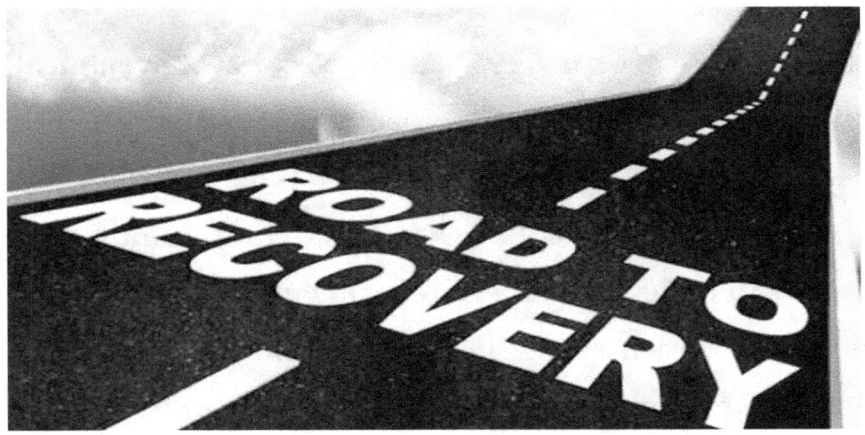

In this Chapter, I will discuss the Patient-Centric Benefits for Direct Access.

Having Quick and Convenient Options for Care

What is it like to be a direct access patient and what are the benefits? If you are experiencing pain, it's no joke. The majority of people who experience pain will typically think of applying an ice pack, popping some medications, buying a brace or immobilizer, or if it's severe enough, heading over to the local urgent-care center. These frequently used "home remedies" or trips to Urgent Care, are often not the best choice for pain. Convenience is crucial. It's the #1 reason why consumers make decisions. You want something quick and easy! If you want something better than a home remedy, direct access to physical therapy will be convenient in these ways:

- Being Nearby
- The Business is Open
- Easy to Get To
- Quick Access to Care (often Same or Next Day Appointment)
- Initiate Treatment Right Away and Feel Better

No Longer Having to Educate Physicians about Physical Therapy in order to Get a Referral (Prescription)

In many cases, consumers, like you, are already educated on the benefits of physical therapy. This could be because you were a patient at some point, or had a friend or family member who received physical therapy in the past, who then told you about it. In my experience, many of my patients have told me they had to go to their physician and actually ask, or even "beg" for a referral

CHAPTER 4

(prescription) to physical therapy. Many of my patients were annoyed that their doctor did not suggest physical therapy first. It's important to understand that with direct access, consumers (patients) won't have to jump through these hoops to gain access to care that they need. It's obvious that when you have pain from an injury, or you are restricted by loss of function due to a disease or disability, physical therapy is often times the best choice for recovery.

Unfortunately, many physicians (other than orthopedists) know very little about physical therapy treatment options and the benefits of physical therapy. Thus, they make very few referrals to physical therapy for their patients. In fact, many patients go without physical therapy because they don't know or have preconceived notions about what physical therapists do.

Direct access allows and encourages patients to become more actively engaged in their own health care decision-making and to proactively address health care concerns before they become real issues and very costly.

Having the Freedom of Choice (Chiropractor vs. Physical Therapist, etc.)

Consumers (patients) benefit from direct access to physical therapy because it eliminates the need for a gatekeeper (physician). This puts the patient more in control of their care, gives them more choices among healthcare providers, reduces delays in receiving beneficial care by eliminating unnecessary office visits to a physician, and ultimately reduces the out-of-pocket costs by avoiding the fees associated with excessive and unnecessary physician office visits.

Direct access laws allow consumers to make their own choice about which healthcare professional they want to see. Before direct access, consumers had a variety of options, such as: chiropractors, massage therapists, acupuncturists, pain management specialists, etc. Physical therapists weren't even on the list and are arguably more qualified to treat the patient. Direct access levels the playing field and gives consumers freedom of choice.

Direct Access: "The Choice Is Yours!"

Ability to Select Your Own Physical Therapist (Not the Physician's Choice)

Some patients still believe that treatment must be provided by a PT associated with that physician's office. This still confuses people. Patients have always been free to see whichever physical therapist they wanted. Yet, it's still commonplace to see physicians using prescription pads from one particular group of physical therapists. Physicians still write orders for physical therapy on one or two of their favorite physical therapy group's pads. As we all know, some physicians are "wined and dined" by certain physical therapy practices in order to get these physicians to refer patients to their practice. Even though "wined and dined" is really not legal, it usually happens in the form of a free lunch, golf outing or tickets to a show. There are physicians who actually have a financial stake or some form of ownership in physical therapy practices, which makes their allegiance to their own physical therapy practice quite obvious. Not all physicians accept these offers or marketing tactics; and the ones that don't generally try to rely on their patient's feedback in order to rate a physical therapy practice and make qualified referrals. However, in all of these cases, physicians are the ones "guiding" their patients on which physical therapist to see.

With direct access that is not the case anymore. Patients can skip seeing these physicians and go right to see a physical therapist of their own volition. Then the patients are able to "comparison shop" physical therapists to find the one that is best for them.

Finding a physical therapy practice that is familiar with direct access laws is imperative. Finding one that has excellent reviews is also important. These physical therapists will be eager to help you, even though you don't have a physician's referral. With just a quick phone call to this physical therapy practice, the front office staff will confirm your insurance and you will be able to see a physical therapist within an hour or two. If the physical therapy practice is knowledgeable about direct access, you won't have to explain why you didn't see a physician first, and they won't be looking for a prescription either. This will be, by far, the best healthcare customer service experience that you ever had. This will typically be the case, when the physical therapist is the first line of care. They know that you haven't seen anyone prior to them, and they will likely be very compassionate, good at listening, and knowledgeable. In Chapter 7, I'll elaborate on how to select a quality direct access physical therapy practice.

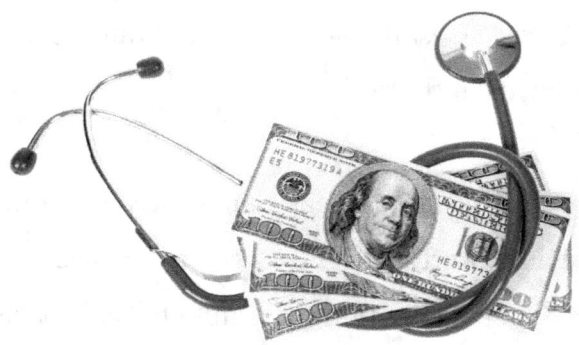

Allocating Your Own Health Care Dollars

Patients are carrying a higher percentage of their health care costs each year. Direct access allows patients to determine how they will allocate their valuable health care dollars. In essence, direct access is similar to buying a product directly from the manufacturer, instead of at a retail store level. In the past, patients were required to go to a retail store (Physician's Office) and pay a higher fee, in order to get the product that they wanted (Physical Therapy), even though the manufacturer (Physical Therapist) had the product that they desired for a lower price. This type of access to physical therapy was only benefiting the physicians and not the patient. This mandatory visit to a referring physician imposed a personal and financial burden on the patient and added an economic burden on the healthcare system as a whole. Access, choice and competition is good for the economy, and in this case, for the patient who needs physical therapy.

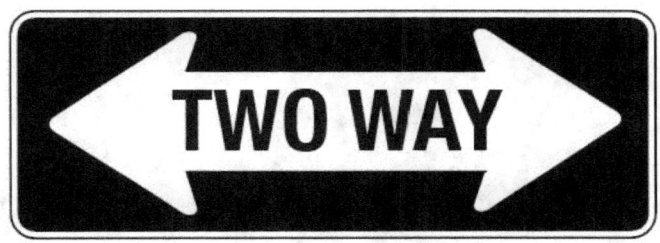

Collaboration is Now a Two-Way Street

Direct access will provide a two-way collaboration model of practice between physical therapists and physicians. Historically, it was a one-way referral model, physician to physical therapist. More recently, physical therapists seeing direct access patients, can suddenly refer to physicians much more than they used to. This is in order to get their patients the best line of care, i.e. when patients can benefit from radiological studies (such as x-rays), medications and/or surgical intervention. Physical therapists are highly qualified to assess and evaluate a patient to determine if physical therapy is appropriate, or if the patient needs the expertise of a physician or other healthcare provider. Physical therapists would coordinate their care with the physicians that were most suited to address the needs of the patient, for example: pain management specialists, orthopaedic surgeons or neurologists, etc. It's sort of a role reversal, but with better intentions of coordinating a patient's care. The referral requirement (in the physical therapy practice act) has created a push for a higher level of mutual respect between physician and physical therapist, and hopefully a deeper understanding of their complementary roles in patient care.

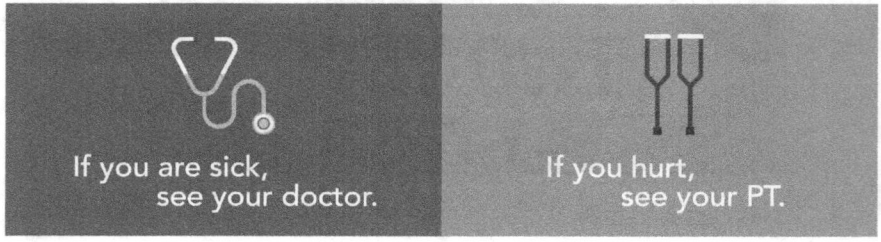

Positive Effects from the "Physical Therapist / Patient" Model

The "physician/patient" model is typically one where the patient sees the physician every few weeks or every few months to follow up. Unlike this model, the "physical therapist/patient" model has a more frequent plan of care, where the patient sees the physical therapist 2 - 3 times a week, over a period of weeks. This allows physical therapists, who are well-educated within the medical model, to be well-positioned to identify medication side-effects or note harmful changes in the patient's condition that might have occurred between physician visits. Physical therapists would be more likely to identify these potential risk factors.

Being Able to Get an Annual Check-Up of Your Musculoskeletal System

Finally, another consumer benefit of Direct Access to Physical Therapy is the patient's ability to come in for an "Annual Check-Up". Primary Care Physicians (PCPs) utilize annual check-ups to evaluate a patient's medical status. Dentists use annual check-ups to evaluate dental health. Optometrists use annual check-ups to evaluate eye sight, and so on. Annual Check-Ups can save billions of healthcare dollars each year by catching early signs of disease and monitoring risk factors for more serious health conditions including: cardiovascular issues, cancers or diabetes, etc. The purpose of an annual check-up in physical therapy would be to evaluate a patient's musculoskeletal function and look for signs of pain, inflammation, lack of mobility, weakness, balance problems and functional limitations in activities of daily living (ADLs).

Many Physical Therapists are now starting to offer free workshops to the general public, to provide people with information on specific injuries or diseases, and to open up channels to discuss ways to prevent and handle the issues. Workshops will teach consumers valuable information on matters such as: low back pain and sciatica, balance and fall prevention, throwing and the overhead athlete, golfer's injury prevention and fitness, proper footwear for runners, and a wide range of other topics.

Physical Therapists who offer these educational workshops are often also providing Free Screenings (FS). Free Screens are one-on-one with a physical therapist, where the goal is to determine whether a person would benefit from a PT evaluation, or referral to another healthcare professional. The consumer would learn the next steps to take to get them moving and feeling better. Many workshops and Free Screens are either done at the physical therapy office or on site within the community. Common places to hold a workshop include: Senior Centers, Running Shoe Stores, Golf Courses, Athletic Centers or Gyms, Schools, and Places of Employment, just to name a few. In Chapter 16, there is a Special Invitation for a Free Screen at your local Physical Therapy office.

Chapter 5

The Big-Picture Benefits of Direct Access Physical Therapy

In Chapter 4, we broke down the benefits of direct access to physical therapy into two distinct categories:

Patient-Centric Benefits: Benefits that deal with the individual consumer's choice of convenience and level of control.

Global Benefits: Benefits that help lower costs and improve healthcare at the local, state, and national levels.

In this Chapter, I will discuss the Global Benefits for Direct Access.

Getting Started Early to Attain Better Outcomes

Over 13 million Americans see their doctor each year for relief from chronic low back pain. The right physical therapy within 14 days of the onset of pain minimizes the average total cost of care by 50%. That's a lot of money back each year!

Low back pain patients who receive physical therapy immediately after the pain begins and adhere to their treatment plan spend

$3,000 a year in associated healthcare costs. Those who delay receiving physical therapy and do not adhere to their treatment plan spend $6,000 per year for all kinds of health care (Fig. 7.).

It was once thought that patients are more likely to stick with a plan when it's physician recommended, because they trust their doctor's expertise. Research shows that is not the case. A 2014 study suggests that patients who received physical therapy through direct access (vs. physician referral) had a higher level of satisfaction and better outcomes at discharge.

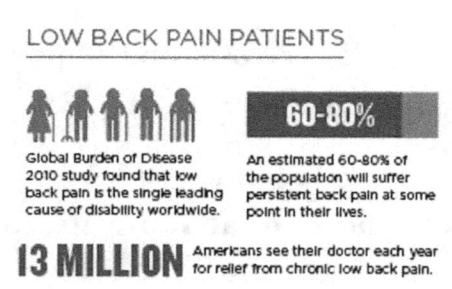

Fig. 7. Low Back Pain Study

Requiring Fewer Physical Therapy Visits than Physician Referred Patients

Earlier research has supported direct access to physical therapists, but the new Health Services Research (HSR) study in Sept 2011, is one of the most comprehensive to date. The HSR study considered 62,707 episodes of physical therapy over a 5-year period, and showed that patients who visited a physical therapist directly for outpatient care (27%) had fewer visits and lower overall costs on average than those who were referred by a physician.

In addition, a 1994 study analyzed 4 years of Blue Cross Blue Shield of Maryland claims data and found that total paid claims for physician referral episodes to physical therapists were 2.2 times higher than the paid claims for direct access episodes (Fig. 8.). In addition, physician referral episodes were 65% longer in duration than direct access episodes and generated 67% more physical therapy claims with 60% more office visits.

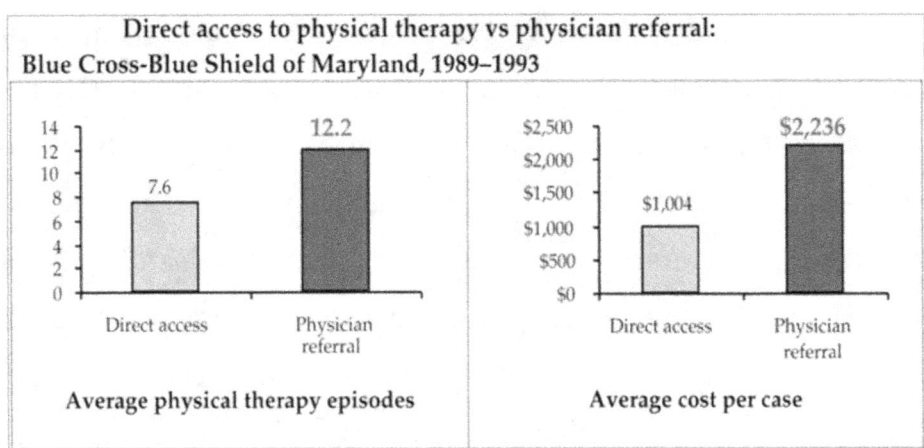

Fig. 8. 1994 Study Data Showing the Benefits of Direct Access

Avoiding Excessive Copays and Other Expenses at the Physician's Office

If a patient is able to see a physical therapist as a "primary" healthcare provider and avoid unnecessary visits to their general practitioner, then total costs for the patient will be lower. Evidence shows that the physician gatekeeper model actually duplicates care. This is ineffective and increases to total cost for the patient.

Less Referrals for Opioid Medications

A trending topic in mid-2017 is the discussion around Opioid Addiction in this country. The Centers for Disease Control (CDC) issued a report in March 2016, which suggested that healthcare professionals must find a better solution to treat chronic pain. Physical Therapy was one of the suggested alternatives to Opioids. Physical therapists treat pain conditions by using modalities such as electrical stimulation, massage, manual therapy, light therapy, low-level laser, ultrasound and hot/cold packs. Even the use of stretching and range of motion exercises can reduce pain. Giving chronic pain patients easier access to physical therapy is one way to reduce the growing Opioid epidemic in this country (Fig. 9.).

CHAPTER 5

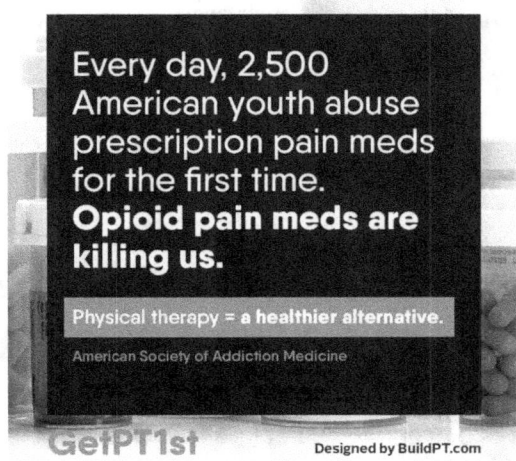

Fig. 9. Advertisement to Help Increase Awareness of Opioid Use in the U.S.

Fewer Number of Emergency Room Visits

The overuse of U.S. Emergency Departments (EDs) is costing this country $38 billion a year in wasteful spending, according to several studies. The cause of these rising costs is due to lack of access to timely primary care services and excessive referrals by primary care physicians themselves. The problem is the wrong care, in the wrong place, at the wrong time (Fig. 10.). EDs are the only place in the healthcare system, where individuals can receive a full range of services, at any time, regardless of their ability to pay. Avoidable ED use is problematic from both a cost and quality standpoint, because of overcrowding, long waits and added stress on the ED staff, which takes away from the patients in need. One strategy to curb ED overuse is direct access to physical therapy for non-urgent musculoskeletal injuries and for patients with chronic disease.

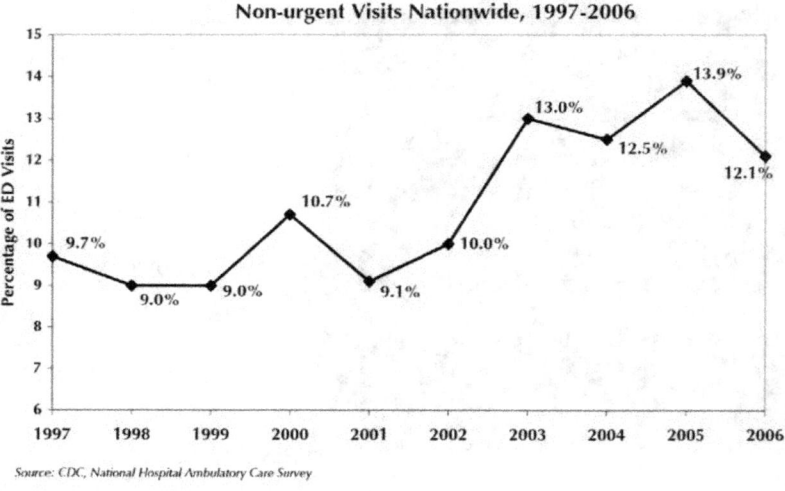

Fig. 10. Graph Shows the Increased of Non-Urgent Emergency Department Visits

Alleviating the Shortage of Primary Care Physicians

According to the American Academy of Family Physicians (AAFP), there is a looming shortage of Primary Care Physicians (PCPs). By 2025, studies estimate a shortfall of between 12,500 and 31,100 PCPs (Fig. 11.). In addition to the shortage of physicians, there is a growing number of older patients who require two to three times the amount of specialty care to treat chronic conditions and age-related illnesses. In addition, there is an aging population of physicians and a shrinking number of students applying to medical schools due to national healthcare reimbursement concerns, rising costs of education, and malpractice expenses.

CHAPTER 5

Dr. Ted Epperly, Director of the AAFP, says doctor shortages lead to poorer health outcomes. Patients often delay care, or in the absence of a general physician, go from specialist to specialist in search of a resolution. Other patients will miss routine prevention and/or management of chronic diseases.

To help alleviate the shortage concerns, there must be a multi-pronged solution. Doctors of Physical Therapy must play the role of primary care provider in addressing musculoskeletal conditions, as they have successfully done for years in the military (See Chapter 6). Physical Therapists are poised, eager to help, and are certainly qualified. Without PTs, there will be a tremendous burden on the healthcare system. Not having enough healthcare professionals to see patients would inevitably clog hospital EDs, worsen patient outcomes and cause patients to go without care, drastically raising the cost of healthcare.

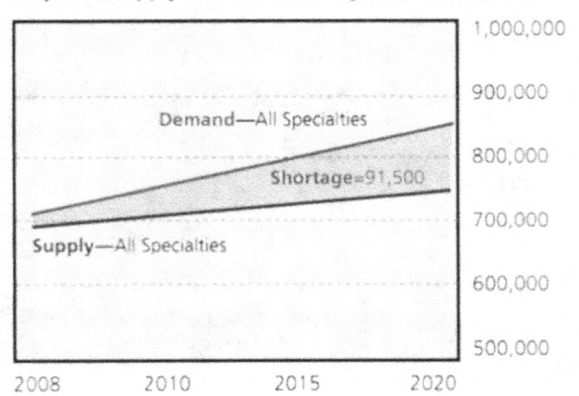

Fig. 11. Graph Showing the Expected Shortage of Physicians within the Next Few Years.

Avoiding Unnecessary Radiological Tests, Medications, Steroid Injections, and Surgery

Research studies show that MRI results of the spine can show many findings, such as: arthritis, decreased disk height, and multiple levels of herniations. These "abnormal" findings are actually normal and due primarily to aging. It is very common to find positive findings on an MRI, yet the patient's diagnosis is different. Therefore, MRIs cannot be relied upon and unless you plan on having surgery the MRI is basically useless. Many people find MRI results to be disconcerting and to take it a step further, receiving an MRI is often times more harmful than beneficial. Early MRIs can lead to poor patient outcomes due to fear-avoidance behaviors, which can intensify symptoms and delay recovery. In addition, using advanced imaging adds roughly $2,500 - $4,800 in costs to a patient's bill (Fig. 12.).

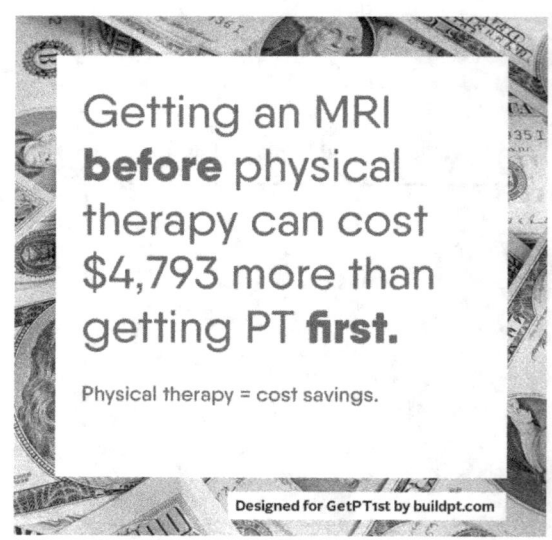

Fig. 12. MRIs are Often Useless and Costly in Many Situations.

CHAPTER 5

X-rays have similar negative value. We all know that x-rays give off harmful radiation. They are also limiting in that they can only image bone. Unless you had a severe fall or collision, i.e. have a bone fracture, an x-ray is not going to present a large amount of information. Physical Therapists are trained to determine if an x-ray or MRI would benefit the patient.

I have to admit, in certain cases surgery is necessary when someone is injured. However, some injuries produce a choice between therapy and surgery, such as a severe Grade III ankle sprain. There are over 27,000 cases of these types of injuries annually and the treatment options are a choice between a "quick" surgery or months of physical therapy. Research shows that patients who choose physical therapy return to work 2-4 times sooner than those that choose surgery. Furthermore, 75% of studies report a faster return to all other pre-injury activity with those who choose physical therapy over surgery. Therapy is often more cost-effective than surgery and is also more likely to help prevent further ankle sprains in the future. While the research process is always ongoing, the general consensus has been that physical therapy works as well, if not better, than surgery (Fig. 13.).

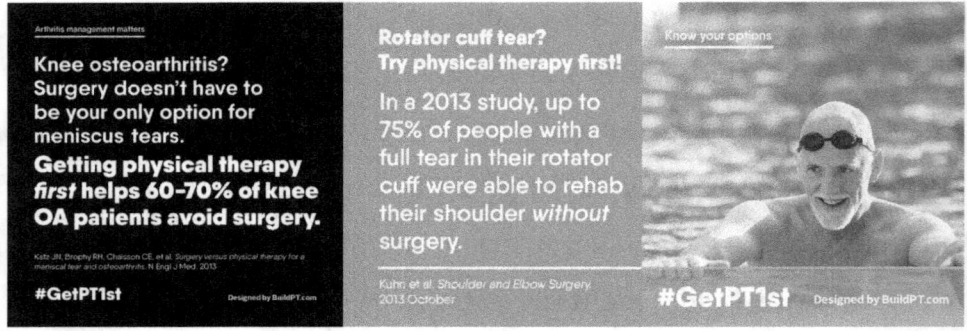

Fig. 13. Getting Physical Therapy First Helps Reduce the Need for Surgery in Many Cases.

Let's delve into the effects of Non-Steroidal Anti-Inflammatory Drugs (NSAIDs), such as Ibuprofen and Naproxen. While they are very helpful at reducing inflammation, they must be used with caution. NSAIDs are associated with frequent and significant side effects that are deleterious to treatment outcomes, including delay in soft tissue and bone healing, renal and liver toxicity, hemorrhagic events, gastric irritation and ulceration, and central nervous system effects. Combining physical therapy with NSAIDs is often the ideal scenario because the patient will likely be able to stop using NSAIDs quicker, thus reducing the risk or severity of side-effects. Recent studies show that NSAIDs are no longer recommended for chronic soft tissue injuries and their use is cautioned with ligament injuries. On a more positive note, there is mounting evidence that exercise and physical activity have anti-inflammatory benefits.

A study published in 2014 has found that a common cause of shoulder pain known as shoulder impingement syndrome can be treated by physical therapy as equally and effectively as steroid injections, with PT being less costly. In the study, steroid injection patients visited their doctor more frequently and requested an additional injection in 60% of the time. The relief from an injection may not last as long, leading to more treatments. Physical therapy involves more patient-clinician contact which allows for range of motion and strengthening exercises, as well as, modalities for pain and a home exercise program. There are also many patients that don't want to have an injection, making physical therapy the best option in many of these situations.

Lower Total Cost of Care
In this age of "healthcare reform", state legislatures continue to seek solutions that will expand access to the health care services the citizens of their state need, while also addressing the growth in health care costs. These health care costs include: physician, testing, special procedures, general hospital, and pharmacy costs. One of the most effective tools for cost control and increased access to easily attainable, yet often overlooked and underutilized by the legislatures, health care is "Direct Access" to services of non-physician healthcare professionals, especially the physical therapist.

DIRECT ACCESS TO PHYSICAL THERAPY

As mentioned in Chapter 1, entry into the profession and practice in the physical therapy profession are stringently regulated by all states. As highly-trained healthcare professionals, physical therapists have a proven track record of effectively treating millions of patients. Physical therapists are well-qualified, both through formal education and clinical training, to evaluate a patient's condition, assess his or her physical therapy needs, and if appropriate, safely and effectively treat the patient. Physical therapists are also well-qualified to recognize when patients demonstrate conditions, signs and symptoms that should be evaluated by other healthcare professionals before therapy is instituted. Physical therapists recognize when it is appropriate to refer patients to these other healthcare professionals for consultation. Therefore, physical therapy should be considered as part of the solution of lowering healthcare costs in the country; with the right care, at the right place, and at the right time.

Chapter 6
The Military has had Direct Access for Years

Our U.S. Military has been utilizing Physical Therapists as Primary Care Providers (PCPs) for patients with musculoskeletal injuries; in other words, using the Direct Access Model, for years.

David G. Greathouse, PT, PhD, ECS, FAPTA, et. al, an Adjunct Professor at the U.S. Army-Baylor University DPT Program, published a study in 2005 on Primary Care Physical Therapy Practice Models which existed in the U.S. Army since 1971. He described a situation in which the U.S. Army was bound by an immense number of patients with neuromuscular problems, a shortage of orthopaedic surgeons, and long delays to see primary care physicians. The mission of the Army Physical Therapist was to serve as independent practitioners (physician extenders) to perform primary care for patients with neuromuscular disorders. While there appeared to be some concerns over the possibility of misdiagnosis or undiagnosis issues, the strengths were the therapists' education and their vast clinical experiences. Based on the need for adequate patient care, the U.S. Army developed protocols for additional continuing education, quality assurance, and eventually a Doctorate Program. Dr. Greathouse's study evaluated the progress of this 40-year endeavor.

DIRECT ACCESS TO PHYSICAL THERAPY

It should be further noted that Physical Therapy Direct Access for the U.S. Army also includes: the ability to order x-rays, bone scans, CT scans and MRIs; the ability to restrict work duties; the ability to prescribe medications, such as analgesics, muscle relaxants and NSAIDs (anti-inflammatory drugs); and the ability to admit a patient and refer to specialty clinics for orthopaedic, neurology, cardiology and/or medical evaluation (Fig. 14.). This does not translate to the civilian world, as we are just beginning to see some States allow PTs to order radiological studies. To date, no State allows PTs to independently prescribe medications to patients.

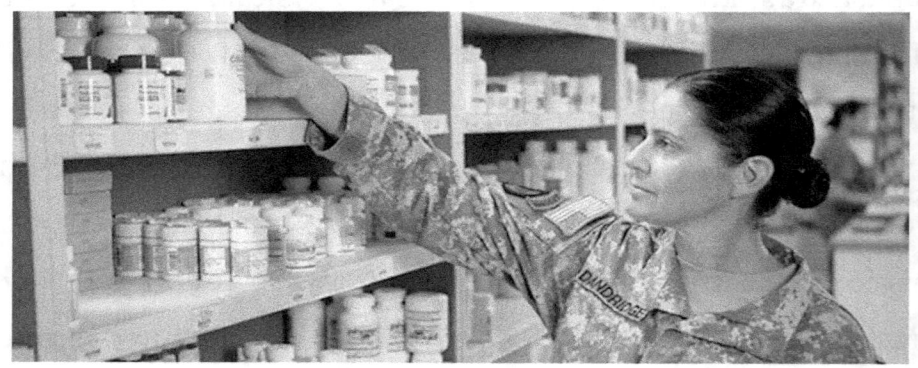

Fig. 14. Military Physical Therapists can Prescribe Medications to Patients.

The U.S. Army determined that the advantages to Physical Therapists having Direct Access included:
- Prompt evaluation and treatment for patients with neuromuscular complaints
- Prompt quality health care

- Decreased sick-call visits
- More appropriate use of physicians
- More appropriate use of PT's education, training and experience.

The Assessment of the U.S. Army's Direct Access Program was astounding! Overwhelming success for 40 years! There was no record of any legal action being brought against any Army PT, as a result of PTs serving in physician extender roles. To this day, they continue to serve in all areas of the Armed Forces, as well as in U.S. Army Medical facilities in California and Utah.

In an article published by the APTA in October 2013, they shared a study out of *"Military Magazine"*, which showed that PTs in the military, acting as Primary Care Providers (PCPs) with unrestricted direct access, provided a better route to recovery than civilian family practice physicians.

- Military PTs used radiology in 11% of case, while family physicians had an 82% usage rate.
- Similarly, Military PTs prescribed medications 24% of the time, while family physicians used medications at a 90% rate.
- Return to Work status was 50% higher for patients who saw the Military PT.

DIRECT ACCESS TO PHYSICAL THERAPY

These findings actually mirror similar efficiencies realized with direct access in the civilian world, according to the author of one report, Lt. Col Troy McGill, PT, MPT, USAF, BSC. When faced with cost containment and an ever-dwindling supply of internists and family practitioners, Lt. Col McGill writes that "PT direct access can help fill this void and give patients the safe and effective care they need in a reasonable time."

The history of Physical Therapy came out of the needs of American Soldiers in WWI. In 1942, Physical Therapists were granted relative military rank. WWII increased the need for PTs and training programs were developed to train physical therapists in the early 1940's. The growth of these programs continued throughout all military deployments around the world. U.S. Military PTs have a proud history of providing medical care during these inherent deployments. This effort has reduced unnecessary medical evacuation of service members with musculoskeletal injuries by approximately 18%. Military PTs are functioning in a primary care direct access role, managing musculoskeletal injuries, and providing evidence-based PT care within a model coined by Colonel Josef Moore called "Sports Medicine on the Battlefield" (Fig. 15.).

CHAPTER 6

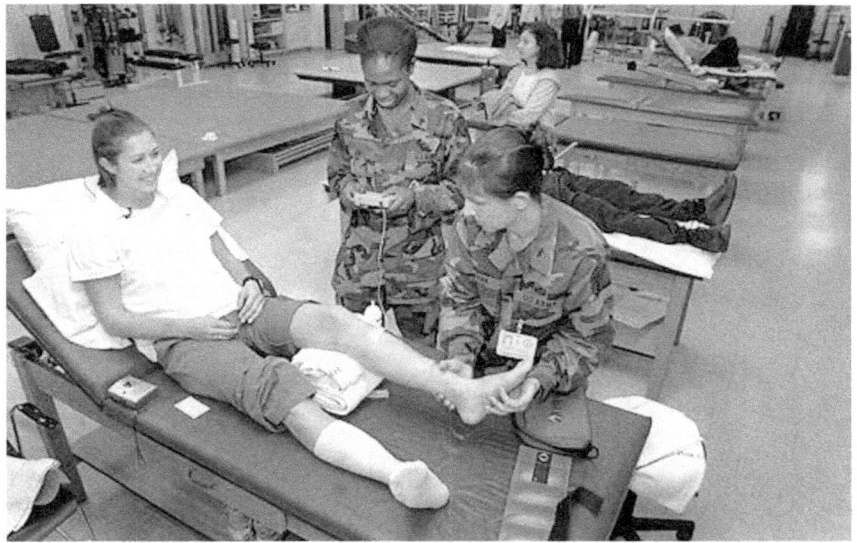

Fig. 15. Military Physical Therapists Providing "Sports Medicine" on the Battlefield.

For many of the Physical Therapists that I know who work in the Military, they will probably never go back to civilian duty, unless Direct Access becomes unrestricted. For them, Direct Access has played an essential role in helping them to provide efficient, safe, and effective treatment to the men and women that serve our country. I'm convinced that a lot of what we learned in the Military, has made an impact on the APTA's vision for the future and now it is up to legislators to make it possible for you, your family, co-workers and friends.

What can you do to help? Check out Chapter 15 for my "Call to Action".

Chapter 7

How to Choose the BEST Physical Therapist for Your Situation

After an injury or surgery, rehabilitation with a physical therapist is often a critical factor on the road to recovery. Most consumers will choose their physical therapist based on proximity to their home or office because physical therapy is typically a weekly commitment and may be for an extended period of time. In most cases, this logic makes sense, as the consideration of convenience is an important factor. Other than convenience, what are the important factors that should go into your decision? Remember, not all Physical Therapy facilities provide the same type or level of care.

It's important for patients to do some research before choosing a location. This might entail talking with your family, co-workers, and friends to see who they would recommend, and then checking on social media sites like Facebook, Google or Yelp for reviews on the locations you are considering.

Choosing the right physical therapist and the right physical therapy practice can make all the difference between failure and success in the rehabilitation process!

DIRECT ACCESS TO PHYSICAL THERAPY

Here are some tips to follow when choosing a Physical Therapy Location:

- Call or visit the facility and ask questions to make sure there are physical therapists with expertise in treating your particular problem.
- Consider how quickly you can get an appointment. If you need to wait more than a week, you may be better off finding a facility where you can start sooner, especially if you have had recent surgery.
- If health insurance is an important consideration for you, make sure the practice accepts your insurance.
- Ask who will be treating you and how much experience the therapist has with your condition.
- Check the location's website for more information about the practice and the physical therapists.
- Before your arrival, the office should have verified your insurance benefits and reviewed any problems with you. Make sure you follow up with the office.
- There should be sufficient parking spaces available close to the location or it should be close to mass transit.
- Good accessibility into the space, preferably on the first floor. Otherwise ramps and elevators should be available.
- The front office staff should be compassionate, knowledgeable, and efficient.
- The office space should be well-lit, organized, and clean.

CHAPTER 7

- Upon arrival, you should be able to quickly and efficiently check-in, ideally with minimal paperwork.
- Consider what the atmosphere is like. You may prefer a more upbeat and energetic facility versus a quiet location. This is personal preference.
- Assess if patients are being treated or if they are sitting around waiting to be treated.

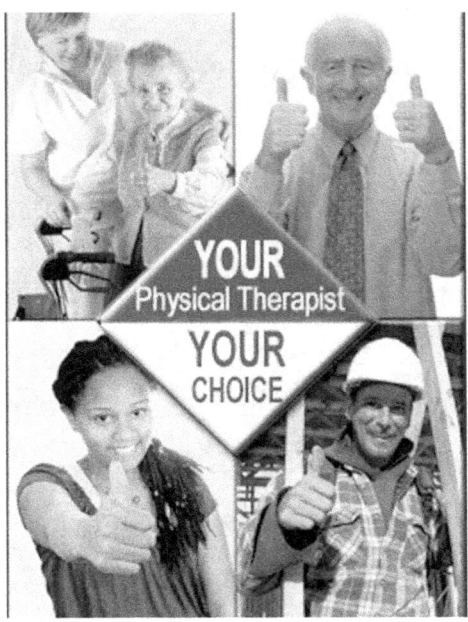

Here are some additional tips to choosing the right Physical Therapist:

- The Physical Therapist's ability to listen goes a long way to understanding your problems and concerns.
- Your appointments should start on time and end within a reasonable period of time.

DIRECT ACCESS TO PHYSICAL THERAPY

- The therapist should be non-judgmental and make eye contact. Your therapist should be someone you could get along with.
- The therapist should be understanding and spend quality time with you.
- You should be asked to complete subjective outcome questionnaires on initial evaluation and at certain periods thereafter.
- You should be able to have a say in your goal setting and plan of care.
- Your treatment plan should have an approximate timeline, so you know what to expect.
- The plan of care should be based on evidence from research readily available to your physical therapist.
- Each visit should be thoroughly explained and dynamically changing (progressive).
- Your treatment program should include prevention training to reduce the risk of re-injury.
- A Home Exercise Program with photos, instructions and number of reps/sets should be provided. An extra bonus would be video instructions with each exercise.
- There should be open lines of communication with your therapist, perhaps via email, text messaging, or through a patient portal.

Chapter 8

The Case for "Think PT First"!

"Think PT First" is my personal initiative to bring awareness to the physical therapy profession and the services that we provide. #ThinkPTFirst!

The "WHEN":
- You lifted a heavy box from the floor a week ago and still have pain when you twist or turn.
- You love to play tennis, but now you can't open a file cabinet or turn a doorknob.
- You played basketball and accidentally fell on your knees. As a result, you are having trouble walking and you are unable to climb the stairs to your bedroom.
- Using a computer is so painful and you can't hold your head up to drive.
- If you are anticipating surgery, studies show that having physical therapy prior to surgery can reduce the time you'll need recovering after surgery.

Do any of these sound familiar? If you have any pain that limits your ability to function fully in your daily life, then you should "Think PT First"! Direct Access to physical therapy may be the right choice for you!

DIRECT ACCESS TO PHYSICAL THERAPY

The "WHY":

- 86% of self-referred patients (i.e. direct access patients) have fewer physical therapy visits than physician referred patients.
- The annual cost for chronic pain is as high as $635 billion a year. That's more than the costs associated with diabetes, heart disease, and cancer combined.
- Employees with back pain are absent from work 4 more days per year than workers without back pain.
- Studies have shown that patients that had PT first, had significantly lower rates of emergency department visits, imaging and opioid prescriptions, as compared to patients that had PT later or never had PT.
- Proper exercise can reduce your risk of reoccurring lower back pain by 25-40%.
- State restrictions on Direct Access has been shown to have significantly increased referrals for imaging and opioid prescriptions.
- Patients who saw a PT first had significantly lower total costs of care compared to those that had PT later or no PT. Total costs including physician, outpatient, hospital, and pharmacy costs.
- Pain affects more Americans than diabetes, heart disease, and cancer combined.

- Lumbar Spinal Stenosis (narrowing of disk spaces), can be treated just as successfully with physical therapy as with surgery; and with 15% fewer complications.
- Common pain conditions (i.e. arthritis, headache, back pain or other musculoskeletal problems) result in $61.2 billion in lower productivity for U.S. workers.
- In a 2013 study, up to 75% of people with a full tear in their rotator cuff were able to rehab their shoulder without surgery.
- Back pain accounts for 10% of primary care physician visits and $86 billion in annual healthcare spending.
- Getting an MRI before physical therapy can cost $4,793 more than getting physical therapy first. Not only that, but MRIs can be misleading. Some findings on an MRI are a normal part of aging and may not be the true cause of your pain.

There are several slogans or hashtags that get consumers' attention, similar to my initiative: #ThinkPTFirst. Some are …. #GetPT1st, #TryPTFirst, #ChoosePT, etc. These represent other groups of physical therapists also trying to spread the word about the benefits of physical therapy! There are obviously some big things happening on social media that are also bringing about awareness, such as: important discussions, blog posts, webinars, workshops, and videos. Don't miss out! Be a part of the conversations and stay informed by tracking some of these popular hashtags.

DIRECT ACCESS TO PHYSICAL THERAPY

The Top 16 Reasons to See a Physical Therapist:
- Low Back Pain and Sciatica
- Post-Surgery
- Headaches and Neck Pain
- Repetitive Sprains or Strains
- Sports Injuries
- Neurological Conditions (Stroke, Parkinson's)
- Joint Pain and Arthritis
- Chronic Pain
- Pregnancy
- Work Related Injuries
- Balance and Vestibular Problems
- Injuries Related to Auto Accidents
- Injury Prevention
- Manage Diabetes and Cardiovascular Conditions
- Manage Women's Health Issues
- Scoliosis and Postural Dysfunctions

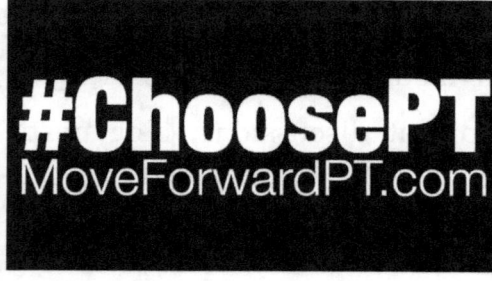
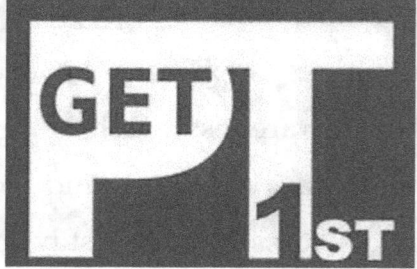

CHAPTER 8

Trending Today: "Physical Therapy – A Safe Alternative to Opioids"

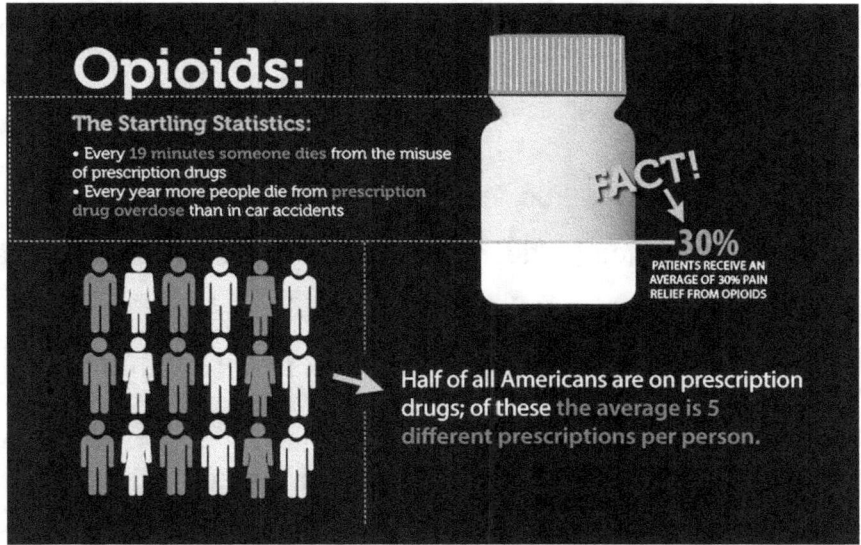

Fig.16. Fact: Patients Receive an Average of 30% Pain Relief from Opioids.

The increased use of opioids for pain management in America has created a national health crisis. Opioid prescription rates have quadrupled since 1999, leading to similar increases in prescription opioid deaths and heroin deaths. Yet, studies show that patients only get 30% relief of pain with Opioid use (Fig. 16.).

In response to America's growing opioid problem, the Centers for Disease Control and Prevention (CDC) released guidelines in March 2016 urging prescribers to reduce the use of opioids in favor of safer alternatives in the treatment of chronic pain. Physical therapy is one of the recommended nonopioid alternatives.

DIRECT ACCESS TO PHYSICAL THERAPY

Here are some reasons to choose physical therapy over Opioid Use:

1. Physical therapists treat pain through movement. Opioids only mask the sensation of pain.

2. Physical therapy "side effects" include improved mobility, increased independence, decreased pain, improved strength, and greater cardiovascular endurance. Opioid side effects include depression, overdose, addiction, and withdrawal symptoms.

3. Physical therapy is effective for numerous conditions and the CDC cited "high quality evidence" supporting exercise as part of physical therapists' treatment for familiar conditions like low back pain, hip and knee osteoarthritis, and fibromyalgia. Opioid effectiveness for long-term pain management is inconclusive in many cases.

It is one thing to teach consumers to "Think PT First", but it is another thing to actually be able to access physical therapy first. Fortunately, Direct Access Laws are heading in the right direction. See Chapter 13 for more information on State Direct Access Laws.

Chapter 9

Are PTs Really Qualified to Deliver Services Without a Physician's Referral?

Two of the major factors discussed when considering direct access to physical therapy services have been:

1. Whether physical therapists are qualified to deliver physical therapy services without the direction and oversight of a physician.

2. Whether there would be an increase in costs for the delivery of physical therapy services. (To be discussed in Chapter 10)

The APTA presents that physical therapists are qualified to deliver services without the necessity of a physician's referral because physical therapists recognize the parameters associated within their scope of practice.

According to Wikipedia, the use of the title doctor by physical therapists and other non-physician healthcare professionals is controversial. In a letter to *The New York Times*, the president of the American Physical Therapy Association responded: "To provide accurate information to consumers, the American Physical Therapy Association has taken a proactive approach and provides clear guidelines for physical therapists regarding the use of the title "Doctor." These guidelines state that physical therapists, in all clinical settings, who hold a Doctor of Physical Therapy degree (DPT) shall indicate they are physical therapists when using the title "Doctor" or "Dr," and shall use the titles in accord with jurisdictional law."

The DPT degree has been described by critics as an example of "credential creep" or degree inflation in *The Chronicle of Higher Education.* Citing concerns that the DPT and similar professional doctorates in areas such as occupational therapy do not meet the standards of traditional doctorate degrees. Critics question whether the rigor of the physical therapy curriculum and the current scope of practice warrant the conferral of a professional degree similar to that characteristic of medicine, dentistry, or nursing.

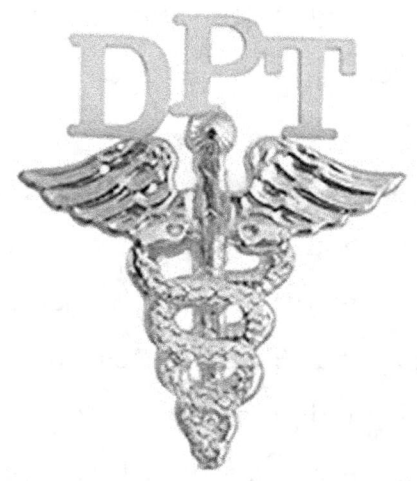

CHAPTER 9

Proponents, myself included, counter the critics by saying that the new curriculum for the doctorate program has far exceeded that of the previous baccalaureate and master's level PT programs. As a leader in the field of physical therapy, Marilyn Moffat, PT, PhD, DPT, FAPTA noted, the previous master's and baccalaureate curricula rival that of most other professional's doctoral programs and these curricula often require more than the typical 72 credits mandated for a doctoral degree in other fields. Released in 2000, the Fact Sheet from the APTA reported that the mean number of credits required for the professional phase of the earlier baccalaureate program was 83.0 credits and that the typical master's degree program required 95.5 credits. As of 2009, the typical number of prerequisite credits was 114.2 and the total number of professional credits was 116.5 for a total of 230.7 credit hours. This is well in excess of the typical 72 professional credits mandated for a doctoral degree in other fields. Additional credit hours may be earned in residency and fellowship programs as well.

A study by, Threlkeld et al. suggests that the scope of existing physical therapy curricula already matches and exceeds that of a professional doctorate, further submitting that students of a well-defined DPT program will have earned the right to be recognized with the doctoral title.

Furthermore, there was a recent Clinical Diagnostic Accuracy (CDA) study comparing Physical Therapists (PT), Orthopaedic Surgeons (OS), and Non-Orthopaedic Physicians (NOP), and their ability to provide an accurate diagnosis as compared to MRI findings. The study revealed that Physical Therapists had a CDA score of 74.5%, Orthopaedic Surgeons scored 80.8%, and Non-Orthopaedic Physicians scored 35.4% (Fig. 17.). The study concluded that Physical Therapists and Orthopaedic Surgeons had a similarly high clinical diagnostic accuracy on patients with musculoskeletal injuries, which was significantly greater than the Non-Orthopaedic Physicians.

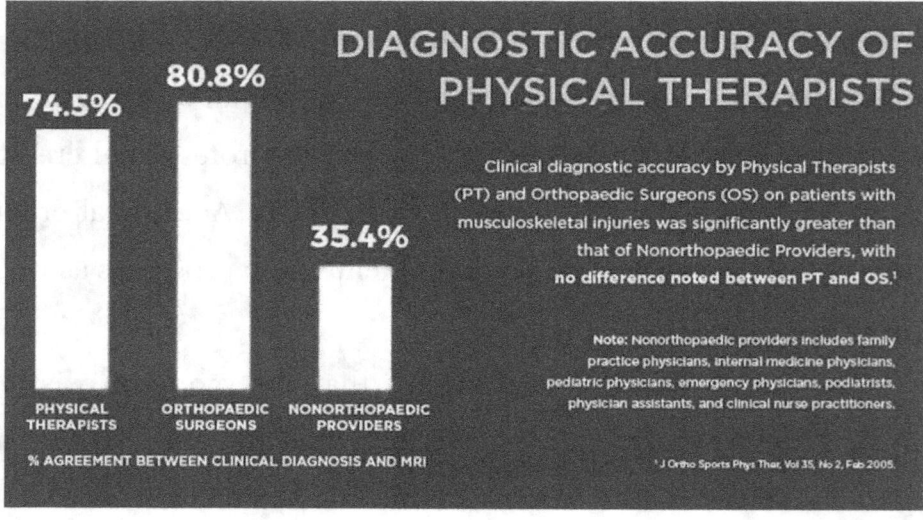

Fig. 17. Physical Therapists and Orthopaedic Surgeons Have Virtually the Same Ability to Diagnose Musculoskeletal Injuries.

Chapter 10

Will There Be an Increase in Healthcare Costs with Direct Access?

In 2015, U.S. Healthcare spending reached $3.2 trillion, or $9,990 per person. The coverage expansion that began in 2014, as a result of in the Affordable Care Act, continued to have an impact on the growth of healthcare spending in 2015. Additionally, faster growth in total health care spending in 2015 was driven by stronger growth in spending for private health insurance, hospital care, physician and clinical services, and the continued strong growth in Medicaid and retail prescription drug spending. Physical Therapy is less than 4% of the total spending in the U.S. (Fig. 18.).

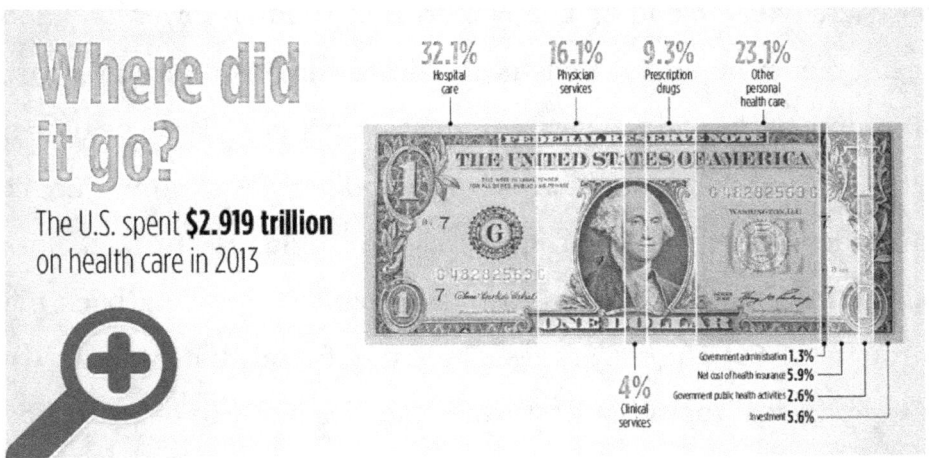

Fig. 18. Physical Therapy Costs are only 4% of Overall Healthcare Costs

DIRECT ACCESS TO PHYSICAL THERAPY

The study by the Health Care Cost Institute (HCCI) suggests that having direct access to physical therapy services may lead to decreases in health care utilization and costs, especially in opioid prescription, Emergency Department (ED) visits, and imaging. The type and extent of the physical therapy access restrictions within state law may affect the amount of health care utilization and cost savings. Given the findings of this study and others, States should consider reviewing their laws that restrict direct access to physical therapy services.

The HCCI study reports that individuals with lower back pain who received physical therapy had reduced healthcare costs when compared to patients who visited another provider first. Patients who visited a physical therapist at the beginning of their treatment were less likely to end up in an emergency room. A lower likelihood of emergency department visits also decreases hospitalization costs. Since low back pain is a very common occurrence in the healthcare setting and a likely contribution to disability, these findings are key to reducing medical spending across the industry. In fact, $90.6 billion in direct healthcare costs are spent on treating back pain throughout the United States. The study found that patients who saw a physical therapist first were also less likely to be prescribed a painkiller when compared to others who saw a different type of clinician. The policy briefly emphasizes that visiting with a physical therapist first will reduce the use of costly healthcare

CHAPTER 10

services and thereby cut spending.

"The findings from this study suggest that seeing a physical therapist as the first point of care compared to seeing a physical therapist at a later point in time (or not seeing a PT) reduces utilization of potentially costly services," as per the Health Care Cost Institute Study (Fig. 19.).

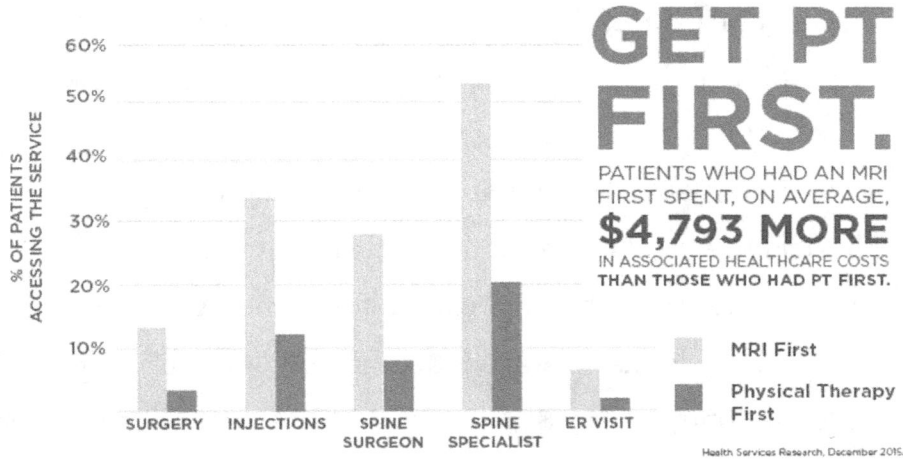

Fig. 19. Evidence that Healthcare Costs will be Lower When Physical Therapy is Provided First.

The APTA reported on a study done by Jean Mitchell of Georgetown University and Gregory de Lissovoy of Johns Hopkins University, wherein the authors found there were more physical therapy claims billed when the services were referred by a physician as compared to fewer claims billed when the physical therapist was working under a direct access scenario. This realization is further supported by the Department of Health and Human Services' Office of Inspector General's (OIG) report from May 2006. The OIG report found approximately 91% of physical therapy services billed by physicians to Medicare beneficiaries in the first 6 months of 2002 did not meet program requirements, which resulted in improper payments of approximately $136 million. Thus, it appears physical therapy services may be over utilized by other healthcare practitioners who have the ability to bill for services under physical therapy codes.

In another study by Mitchell and Lissovoy, the total paid claims for physician referral episodes to physical therapists was 123% or 2.2 times higher than the paid claims for Direct Access episodes. The total paid claims averaged $2,236 for "physician referral" episodes, as compared to $1,004 for Direct Access (self-referred) episodes. When expressed in terms of actual reimbursements, the difference in total paid claims per episode was $1,232. This is real money that patients and payers will be saving.

This data analysis supports the idea that physical therapists under direct access would not abuse the reimbursement system. In short, research shows that health care costs will be lower with direct access to physical therapy and there is no evidence to suggest that an increase in health care costs is immanent.

Chapter 11

The Argument from Medical Professionals and Chiropractors on Direct Access to Physical Therapy

Chiropractic and medical organizations consistently attempt to point out the risk to patients going to physical therapy without a referral and often make inaccurate statements about a Physical Therapist's ability to diagnose pathologies. The caveat is that all professional organizations have the right and responsibility to advocate for patient/public safety and well-being, so the fact that these organizations are challenging physical therapist's initiatives is appropriate.

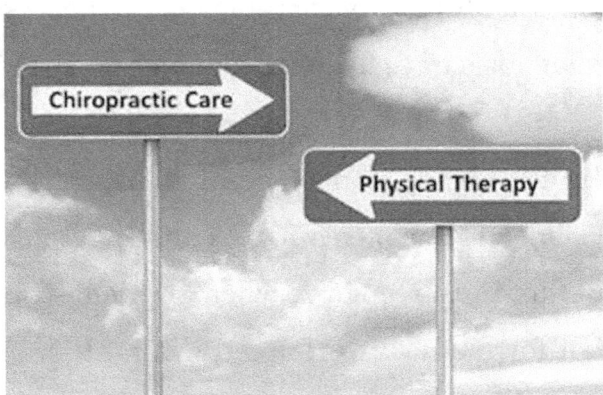

Some of the issues raised by opponents to Direct Access include: patient safety, the professional education of a physical therapist, and whether or not a physical therapist is able to diagnose patients.

DIRECT ACCESS TO PHYSICAL THERAPY

Let's look at some of these issues below:

Patient Safety: Patient/public safety is no less a concern for physical therapists, than as compared to any medical or chiropractic professional. This priority for patient safety is clearly noted in the APTA Standards of Practice, the Code of Ethics, and the Guide to Professional Conduct. In addition, most state's physical therapy practice acts have language, such as "Duty to Refer" if the physical therapist has reasonable cause to believe that symptoms or conditions are beyond the scope of their practice.

Professional Education: Medical Screening is a curriculum content area that has been significantly enhanced over the years, to teach physical therapists how to recognize findings that are unusual and inappropriate for physical therapy management. Textbooks on the topics of pathology, medical screening and differential diagnosis have been in existence for over 15 years.

Medical Diagnosis: It is not necessary for physical therapists to make a "Medical" Diagnosis for a condition such as cancer or infection, but they must recognize when a patient should be referred to a physician for medical workups. Physical therapists routinely collect patient health history about illnesses, surgeries, medication use, etc., and see the patient more frequently, allowing them to often see the bigger picture of a patient's condition sooner than other medical professionals would.

CHAPTER 11

A question worth exploring is: How does a Physical Therapist's knowledge in musculoskeletal medicine compare to that of a physician's?

In a study by Freedman and Bernstein, clinical knowledge was assessed in basic nonsurgical musculoskeletal medicine among 85 physicians during their first week of their internship following graduation from medical school, using a standardized examination. The mean score was just under 60%, with only 18% of physicians scoring above a level determined by orthopaedic program directors, as the minimum threshold necessary to establish competency in musculoskeletal medicine in the primary care setting. In a comparable study, Matzkin et al, demonstrated similar suboptimal levels of knowledge in musculoskeletal medicine among medical students, residents, and virtually all physician specialists except for orthopedists.

Physical Therapists, J. Childs and J. Whiteman, set out to replicate the Freedman and Bernstein study using both physical therapy students nearing graduation and practicing physical therapists. The study looked at 174 physical therapy students from 12 randomly selected educational programs and 182 practicing physical therapists. The physical therapists and physical therapy students were then asked to complete the same examination administered by Freedman and Bernstein and Matzkin, assessing knowledge in managing musculoskeletal conditions.

The results showed that practicing physical therapists demonstrated higher levels of knowledge in managing musculoskeletal conditions than medical students, physician interns, residents, and all physician specialists except for orthopaedic surgeons. Furthermore, practicing physical therapists who were board certified in orthopaedic or sports physical therapy, achieved significantly higher scores and passing rates than their non–board-certified colleagues. The results also showed a 67% pass rate among practicing physical therapists, which is greater than the 60% pass rate of their physician counterparts. Physical therapy students also performed better than all physician groups except for orthopaedic surgeons.

Many consumers still rely on medical doctors to have the right knowledge of musculoskeletal conditions to make a necessary referral to a physical therapist, despite studies showing that they may have less than the preferred knowledge base. Consequently, this suggests why educated consumers were often the one's approaching their general practitioners and primary care physicians for approval to go see a physical therapist.

There is also the question: Are medical doctors and surgeons, chiropractors and pharmaceutical companies' motives really

CHAPTER 11

for patient safety? As noted in a paper called, "The Future of Chiropractic Revisited: 2005 – 2015", Physical Therapists are considered the primary economic threat to the future of chiropractic practice, which implies more concern for their financial situation.

Nationally, many states have had some form of direct access to physical therapy for many years and there is no evidence of any adverse patient events. As mentioned earlier in Chapter 6, physical therapists in the U.S. Army have been utilizing unrestricted direct access, in addition to being able to refer for x-rays and MRIs, as well as prescribe medications all without incident. Overall, there has not been a single case of patient injury or an adverse event directly correlated with direct access policies. While there has been evidence of increased liability cases for physical therapists, this may be related to an increasing average age of the population, leading to the rising number of patients seeing a physical therapist.

The physical therapy profession understands the responsibility associated with the privilege of seeing patients without a physician referral. Steps have long been taken to make sure we have appropriate patient safety practice standards, the regulatory mechanisms set up to oversee physical therapy practice, and the education model established to prepare competent physical therapy practitioners. The result will be more physical therapist and physician communication, not less.

DIRECT ACCESS TO PHYSICAL THERAPY

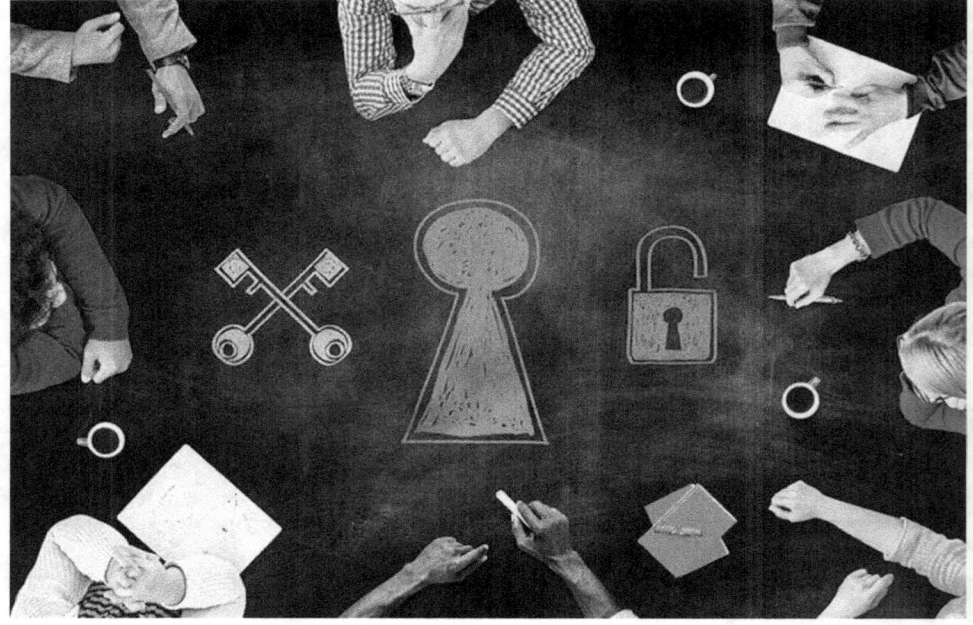

Fig. 20. A Collaborative Relationship between Physical Therapists and Physicians is Vital.

Both physical therapists and physicians must be vigilant about creating a mutual respect for, and deep understanding of, their complementary roles in patient care. With that understanding, direct access to physical therapy services (without requirement of a physician referral) does not alter that relationship. It merely allows the collaboration to be initiated by the physical therapist at a point in the physical therapy episode of care that is most beneficial to the patient, and most cost-effective for the healthcare system (Fig. 20.).

CHAPTER 11

With physical therapists, it's not about putting another profession out of business or into duress. There are plenty of patients to go around, and direct access to physical therapy will only help physicians focus on the patients that truly need them, i.e. ones with medical and surgical needs. Physical therapists will be referring to physicians, instead of the other way around, hence a much more efficient system of healthcare. While I can't speak for physicians and chiropractors, I would strongly believe that they want to have more patients they can actually treat and help in their offices, rather than people just looking for unnecessary testing and prescription drugs. There is huge potential for everyone to benefit from direct access.

Chapter 12

Medicare Beneficiaries – Are You Able to Get Direct Access to Physical Therapy Services?

As of 2005, per the Medicare Benefit Policy Manual, Medicare beneficiaries may seek physical therapy services without seeing a physician or obtaining a referral. Sounds pretty good, right!? We know it wouldn't be Medicare if it was truly that simple.

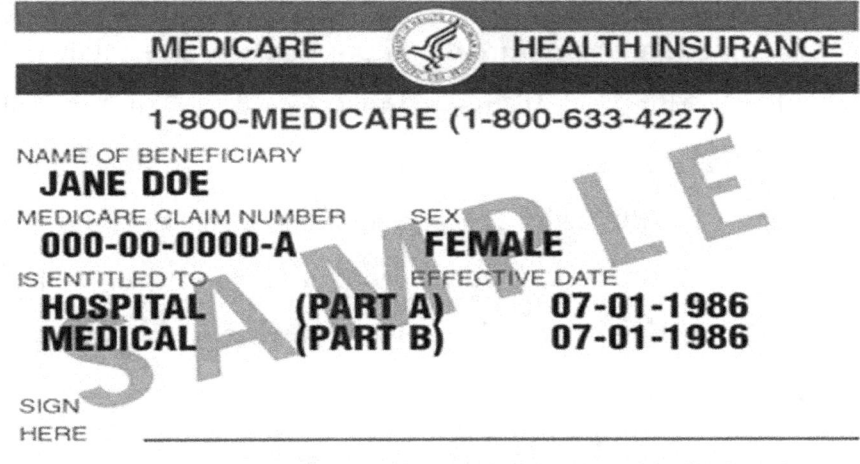

Always comply with your state's laws regarding direct access. You can review state laws online, under the Physical Therapy Practice Act for your state. In general, Medicare does not require patients to obtain prescriptions from physicians for physical therapy services. However, physical therapists must develop a plan of care (POC)

DIRECT ACCESS TO PHYSICAL THERAPY

for every Medicare patient, and, a physician or non-physician practitioner (NPP) must certify that POC within 30 days of the initial physical therapy visit. Medicare does not require the patient to actually visit the certifying physician or NPP, although that physician or NPP may require a visit. For the record, the POC must at minimum include: a diagnosis, long term treatment goals, and the type, quantity, duration and frequency of the physical therapy services.

When a physician or NPP certifies a POC, he or she must sign and date it. Stamped signatures are not allowed. If the physician or NPP gives verbal certification, he or she must provide a signature within 14 days of that verbal notice. In addition, the physical therapist must recertify the POC within 90 calendar days from the date of the initial treatment or if the Medicare patient's condition evolves in such a way that the physical therapist must revise long-term goals, whichever comes first.

Keep in mind, that Medicare can change its policy and it is always best to check with Medicare directly.

Chapter 13

The Latest Issues That Affect YOUR Rights to Direct Access Physical Therapy Services

As of January 1, 2015, all 50 States, the District of Columbia and the US Virgin Islands allow patients to seek some level of treatment from a physical therapist without a prescription or referral from a physician, according to the American Physical Therapy Association (APTA).

Unfortunately, there are still some states that arbitrarily place restrictions on the number of visits allowed without a prescription or referral from a physician, have limited types of patient populations, or only allow certain types of treatments under their state's direct access law (Fig. 21.). It is the APTA's position that these restrictions do not recognize the high level professional training and expertise of the licensed physical therapist, nor do they serve the needs of those patients who require physical therapy but whose care is unnecessarily interrupted by these restrictions.

DIRECT ACCESS TO PHYSICAL THERAPY

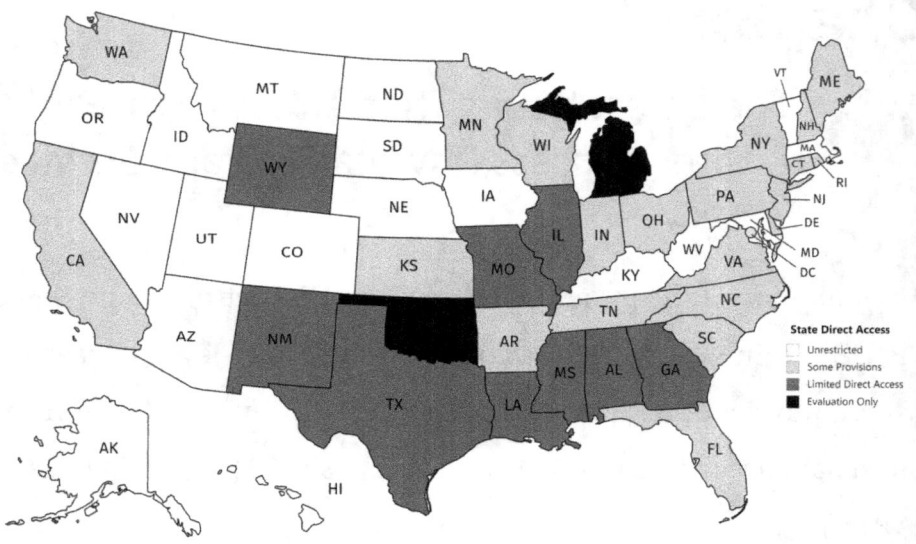

Fig. 21. Patchwork of Different Levels of Direct Access Law throughout the U.S.

The story of Direct Access is still unfolding. It is the ongoing work of PTs across the country to make direct access a reality in the face of stiff opposition. With Direct Access established in some form in every State, APTA's focus has shifted from the quantity of states and localities with direct access, to the quality of those jurisdictions' direct access laws.

"While the ultimate objective is unrestricted direct access in every state and locality, the immediate goal is to remove those barriers to access that are causing the biggest problems for patients.", according to Angela Shuman, Director of State Government Affairs at APTA. The priority, in other words, is to have direct access laws in place in every jurisdiction that work for both patients and PTs in those locations.

"The profession is getting there", Shuman emphasizes, "but that isn't to say that the road to date has been smooth, or that the stretch ahead is obstacle-free".

As of June 2016, here is a look at the Level of Patient Access to Physical Therapy, by State:

Limited Patient Access (6 States)
For certain patient populations or under certain circumstances (i.e. treatment restricted to patients with a previous medical diagnosis or subject of a previous physician referral).

Alabama
Missouri
Illinois
Texas
Mississippi
Wyoming

DIRECT ACCESS TO PHYSICAL THERAPY

Patient Access with Provisions (26 States, DC, and U.S. Virgin Islands)

Access to evaluation and treatment with some provisions such as a time or visit limit.

Arkansas	New Jersey
California	New Mexico
Connecticut	New York
Delaware	North Carolina
District of Columbia	Ohio
Florida	Oklahoma
Georgia	Pennsylvania
Indiana	Rhode Island
Kansas	South Carolina
Louisiana	Tennessee
Maine	Virginia
Michigan	Washington
Minnesota	Wisconsin
New Hampshire	

CHAPTER 13

Unrestricted Patient Access (18 Total)

No restrictions or limitations whatsoever for treatment absent a referral.

Alaska	Montana
Arizona	Nebraska
Colorado	Nevada
Hawaii	North Dakota
Idaho	Oregon
Iowa	South Dakota
Kentucky	Utah
Maryland	Vermont
Massachusetts	West Virginia

For more information on Direct Access Laws in your State, go to your State Government Website or contact your State Legislators. You can also check the www.APTA.org/Chapters website for a list of state chapters.

Chapter 14

"We The People"...Have Rights!
State Policymakers Should Take Action

Every State, the District of Columbia, and the U.S. Virgin Islands have all recognized the safety and benefits of direct access to physical therapy by removing from their statutes, all or some of the referral requirements or provisions for a physical therapy evaluation and treatment (see Chapter 13 for an overview of State Policies).

However, a 2013 study revealed that only 35% of policy makers and 16% of physicians were supportive of direct access to physical therapy. While these numbers have certainly improved over the past few years, there is still resistance to the change. Given the positive results of so many studies, it is up to the States to consider reviewing their laws that restrict direct access to physical therapy services.

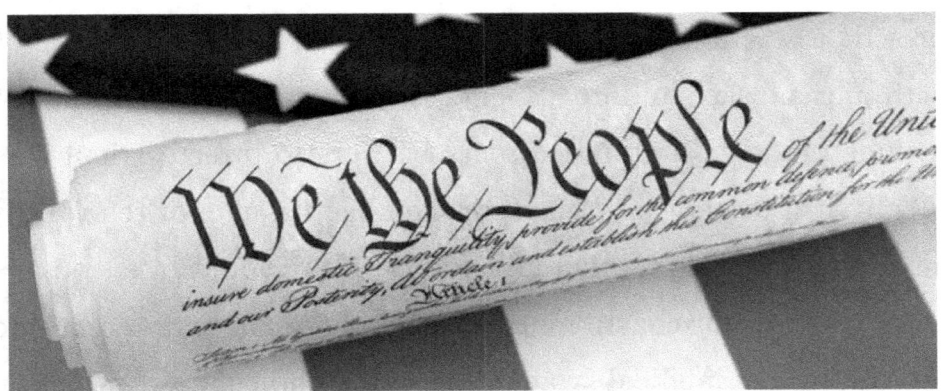

DIRECT ACCESS TO PHYSICAL THERAPY

Direct Access to Physical Therapy is a basic Human Rights issue.

Calling all Constituents (Consumers) in States without Unrestricted Direct Access Laws:

If you live in a State that continues to utilize outdated and unnecessary barriers to patients receiving full access to physical therapy, please consider a movement in your State to reform the laws by contacting your State officials to encourage a change. By amending the physical therapy practice act in your State, everyone who lives there will gain a beneficial entry point into the traditional medical system, increased choice in the selection of a healthcare professional, and access to less expensive and more timely care. In other words, lifting the restrictions on physical therapists and allowing people to have increased access to care, will also free the State from the burden of high cost healthcare.

Calling all State Policymakers:

As a legislator, you can feel confident that physical therapists provide a safe and cost-effective means of treatment for patients with musculoskeletal impairments. If your State laws continue to include outdated and unnecessary barriers to direct patient care by physical therapists, please consider the benefits of reform. By amending the physical therapy practice act in your State, you will be providing your constituents with an additional entry point into the traditional medical system, increased choice in the selection of a healthcare professional, access to less expensive and more timely care, and a simple, yet extremely effective way to meet the goals of increased access and cost containment.

For additional information on direct access, please contact APTA's State Government Affairs Department at 800/999-2782, ext. 3161 or visit www.APTA.org/StateAdvocacy/

Chapter 15

Final Thoughts & How You Can "Pay It Forward"

In Chapters 1 and 2, you learned about the history of physical therapy, the extensive training and the six (6) key principles that guide physical therapists forward. In Chapter 3, you read about Direct Access to Physical Therapy and how it is defined as a form of self-referral; where consumers can get unrestricted access to see a physical therapist without a prescription. I gave the analogy of planning a vacation, and how important getting the most convenient direct flight, with fewest stops and lowest fares, is to the overall experience of an amazing vacation. The "vacation experience" correlates to a consumer's road to recovery, i.e. the path to physical therapy. I've shared how enlightened and amazed people are when they learn how much easier it is to get physical therapy, how it will save them significant time and money, and most importantly, give them better treatment outcomes as compared to other interventions.

In Chapters 4 and 5, many of the consumer's benefits were outlined as they pertained to individual's patient-centric benefits and more global population-based benefits. Here is a simple summary of the Consumer's benefits to having Direct Access to Physical Therapy:

DIRECT ACCESS TO PHYSICAL THERAPY

Patient-Centric Benefits:
- Having Quick and Convenient Options for Care
- No Longer Having to Educate Physicians about Physical Therapy in order to Get a Referral (Prescription)
- Having the Freedom of Choice (Chiropractor vs. Physical Therapist, etc.)
- Ability to Select Your Own Physical Therapist (Not the Physician's Choice)
- Allocating Your Own Health Care Dollars
- Collaboration is Now a Two-Way Street
- Positive Effects from the "Physical Therapist / Patient" Model
- Being Able to Get an Annual Check-Up of Your Musculoskeletal System

Global Benefits:
- Getting Started Early to Attain Better Outcomes
- Requiring Fewer Physical Therapy Visits than Physician Referred Patients
- Avoiding Excessive Copays and Other Expenses at the Physician's Office
- Less Referrals for Opioid Medications
- Fewer Number of Emergency Room Visits
- Alleviating the Shortage of Primary Care Physicians
- Avoidance of Unnecessary Radiological Tests, Medications, Injections, and Surgery

CHAPTER 15

- Lower Total Cost of Care (costs include: physician, testing and special procedures, hospital, and pharmacy costs)

In Chapter 6, I outlined how successful the U.S. Military has been in utilizing direct access to lower costs and provide more efficiencies in health care, and, how the Army has been doing it for over 40 years! In Chapters 7 and 8, I provided helpful tips on how to choose the best physical therapist for your particular situation, and when to "#ThinkPTFirst". Chapters 9 through 12 gave countless examples of evidence that physical therapists have exceptional knowledge and expertise in the musculoskeletal system, and provide the best interventions in many cases above and beyond those of their physician counterparts. According to Chapters 13 and 14, there is still a long way to go in the quest to get unrestricted direct access in every State throughout the nation.

Most importantly and simply put, I feel that it our duty as physical therapists to help people achieve relief from pain and restore function, with the best outcomes, at the lowest cost, and in the least amount of time. I'm optimistic that this book will serve as a vehicle to spread the word to the consumer about the benefits of unrestricted "direct access to physical therapy".

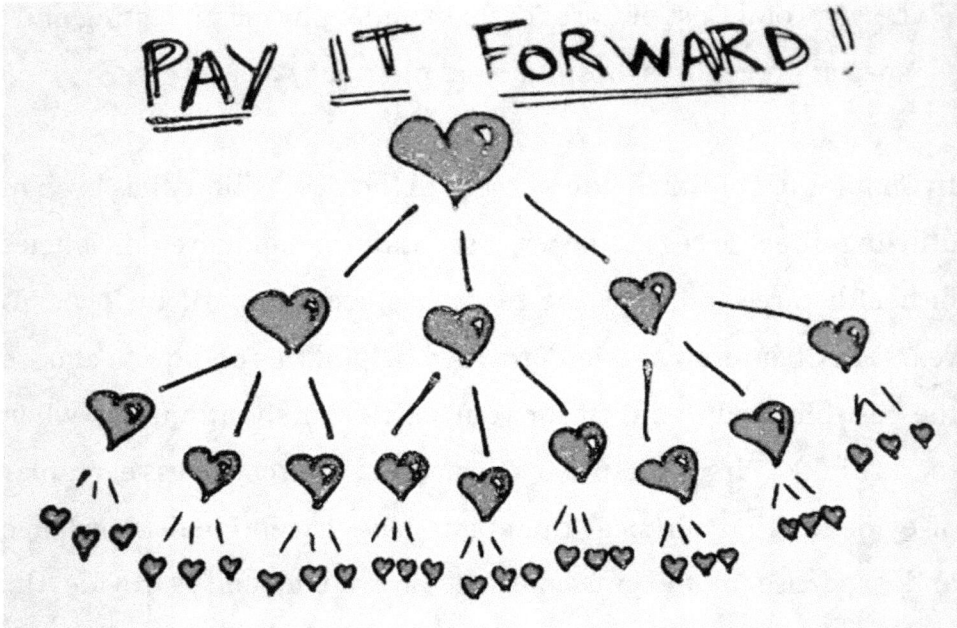

Let's Pay It Forward!

Wrapping this up, I hope you are now as passionate as I am and want to get involved in achieving unrestricted Direct Access to Physical Therapy for everyone, including your co-workers, friends, and family members!

My "call to action" is for everyone who has read this book and taken away at least one or two pearls of information, to pass the book along to someone else who might reap the benefits just like you have! Sort of a "Pay it Forward" movement that I would enjoy seeing as the reward for my efforts in putting this book together for you.

CHAPTER 15

The situation I wrote about in the Preface is the true reason why I wrote this book. It was frustrating having to share information about "Direct Access to Physical Therapy" with one person at a time, with whom, by the way, were patients already sitting in my office. Thankfully, this book gives me an avenue to reach you, many others like you, and people you care about, who will likely benefit from the information I have gathered and the opinions I have shared.

So Please....Pass This Book Along and Pay It Forward!

DIRECT ACCESS TO PHYSICAL THERAPY

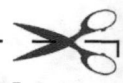

YOUR "FREE SCREEN" OFFER!

Present this page to receive Your Free Screening!

You'll be Spending 20-30 min. with a Licensed Physical Therapist

PT Office – Affix a label here with Business Name, Address, Website & Contact Info**

Your Free Screen Includes:

1. Determining the Basic Cause of Your Pain
2. Learning About Your Treatment Options
3. Finding out if Physical Therapy is Right for You
4. Having Peace of Mind

**Note to PT Office Manager:

For more information on the "Free Screening" Procedure, Contact: Support@DirectAccessToPhysicalTherapy.com

**Note to Physical Therapists (PTs):

Free Screening Laws are different in every State. Please check with your State's Practice Act to determine any restrictions or guidelines.

Chapter 16

Your FREE BONUS for Reading This Book!

If you, or someone you know, is currently suffering from pain, inflammation, stiffness, weakness or any other physical condition, feel free to copy or tear out this page and present it to the physical therapy location listed to the left. This is YOUR free BONUS for reading this book. Exercise your right to Direct Access and see a Licensed Physical Therapist near you!

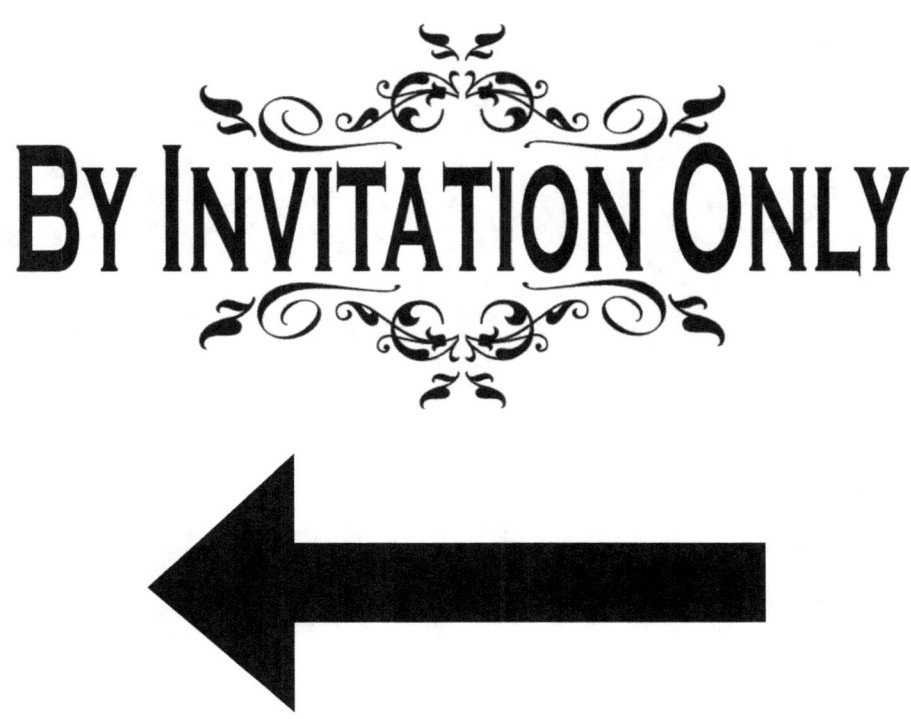

References

A Global View of Direct Access and Patient Self-Referral to Physical Therapy: Implications for the Profession. Phys Ther, April 2013

A History of Manipulative Therapy, Journal of Manipulative Therapy. 2007; 15(3): 165 – 174

A Matter of Urgency: Reducing Emergency Department Overuse. NEHI Research Brief, March 2010

American Physical Therapy Association (APTA) – www.APTA.org Accessed June 2017

B. Murphy, PT and Greathouse, PT, PhD, et. al., Primary Care Physical Therapy Models. Journal of Orthopaedic & Sports Physical Therapy. November 2005

C.A. McCallum and T. DiAngelis, Direct Access: Factors that Affect Physical Therapist Practice in the State of Ohio. Physical Therapy 92(5): 688-706, Feb 2012

C. Bohnett and WebPT, Medicare and Direct Access. Oct 2014

C. Lefferts and WebPT, Direct Access from the Patient's Perspective. June 2015

Clinical Diagnostic Accuracy and MRI of Patients Referred by Physical Therapists, Orthopaedic Surgeons, and Non-orthopaedic Providers. JOSPT, Feb 2005

D. Belk, MD, True Cost of Health Care. www.TrueCostofHealthcare.net Accessed June 2017

Direct Access: The Truth About Seeing a PT First. ProRehab PT, May 2017

Does Unrestricted Direct Access to Physical Therapy Reduce Utilization and Health Spending? Health Care Cost Institute (HCCI) www.healthcostinstitute.org/files/HCCI-Issue-Brief-Unrestricted-Access-to-Physical-Therapy.pdf Accessed June 2017

E. Ries, PT, The State(s) of Direct Access by in Motion. October 2016

H. Ojha, R. Snyder and T. Davenport, Direct Access Compared with Referred Physical Therapy Episodes of Care: A Systematic Review. Phys Ther (2014) 94 (1): 14-30.

J. Childs and J Whitman, Advancing Physical Therapy Practice: The Accountable Practitioner. JOSPT, 2005

J. Giulietti, The History of Physical Therapy. http://www.eugenept.com/history Accessed June 2017

J. Mitchell and Dr. G. de Lissivoy, A Comparison of Resource Use and Cost in Direct Access Versus Physician Referral Episodes of Physical Therapy. Phys Ther, Jan 1997

J. Moore, et.al, The Role of U.S. Military Physical Therapists During Recent Combat Campaigns. Phys Ther (2013) 93 (9): 1268-1275

J. Pendergast, PhD, et. al., A Comparison of Health Care Use for Physician-Referred and Self-Referred Episodes of Outpatient Physical Therapy. Sept 2011

K. Sullivan, et.al., A Vision for Society: Physical Therapy as Partners in the National Health Agenda. Phys Ther 2011; 91 (11): 1664-1672

M. Moffat., Three Quarters of a Century of Healing Generations. Phys Ther (1996) 76:1242 – 1252.

Physical Therapist Practice and the Human Movement System. APTA White Paper, 2015

R. J. Grella, Direct Access to Physical Therapists: An Advocate's Handbook. Practice Repetitions, LLC, Palm Harbor, FL, 2014

R. Scott Ward, Take That Step. Phys Ther (2012) 92 (9): 1230-1234.

Significant Primary Care, Overall Physician Shortage Predicted by 2025. AAAFP, March 2015

S. K. Nicholson, Esq, MBA, PT, The Physical Therapist's Business Practice and Legal Guide. Jones and Bartlett Publishing, 2008

T. Ambury and WebPT, Direct Access: What are the Risks? Oct 2014

T. Davenport, et. al., The Physical Therapist as a Diagnostician: How Do We, Should We, and Could We Use Information About Pathology in Our Practice? Phys Ther (2011) 91 (11): 1694-1695.

The Movement System Brings It All Together. PT in Motion Magazine, May 2016

Threlkeld, AJ, et. al., The Clinical Doctorate: A Framework for Analysis in Physical Therapist Education. Physical Therapy Journal, 1999

W. Boissonnault, Direct Access: Where's the Beef? The Challenge From Chiropractors. AAOMPT Official Newsletter: Articulations, 2006

Book Ordering Information

Individual Consumer: As you hopefully have discovered, "*Direct Access to Physical Therapy: The SECRET Revealed --- How to Relieve Pain & Restore Function WITHOUT Medications, Injections, or Surgery*" was written to present the benefits of self-referral to physical therapy. If you would like to order a copy for a friend or family member or bring a few copies to work or school, please order from the website below.

PT Clinics: This is a great gift to handout or mail to patients immediately following their initial evaluation. The patients will love getting something in the mail from you! The book offers valuable information that patients can share with friends and family. You can also distribute the book at workshops and events. As a reminder, don't forget to affix your Clinic's Contact Information to the Free Screen Offer in Chapter 16.

If you would like to order additional copies of this book, go to: https://www.createspace.com/7210327

Volume discounts are available.
For more information, please contact the author directly at: Support@DirectAccessToPhysicalTherapy.com

www.ingramcontent.com/pod-product-compliance
Lightning Source LLC
Chambersburg PA
CBHW071211240526
45470CB00018B/1712